DISEASE
DATA
BOOK

DISEASE
DATA
BOOK

John Fry
General Practitioner, Beckenham, Kent

Gerald Sandler
Consultant Physician, Barnsley District General Hospital

David Brooks
General Practitioner, Manchester

⊞

Published, in association with
Hastings Hilton Publishers Limited,
by

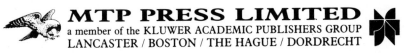

MTP PRESS LIMITED
a member of the KLUWER ACADEMIC PUBLISHERS GROUP
LANCASTER / BOSTON / THE HAGUE / DORDRECHT

Published in association with
Hastings Hilton Publishers Limited, London, by
MTP Press Limited
Falcon House
Lancaster, England

ISBN 0-85200-922-4

Photoset and printed by Redwood Burn Limited,
Trowbridge, Wiltshire

CONTENTS

PREFACE

Here we offer a new approach to understanding and managing common medical conditions. With the needs of our readers in mind we present clearer, more extensive and more expansive views on them.

Traditional medical textbooks are wordy tomes with well worn patterns dealing in set order with 'causes, symptoms and signs, diagnosis and treatment'. They offer formal instant snapshots of diseases.

We have devised an economic synoptic style, and we have endeavoured to give a comprehensive and an on-going long term move picture of each condition and to relate this to the analysis of symptoms and signs, to diagnostic assessment and to management and treatment.

We have selected 22 important conditions and for each have followed the same sequence of questions and answers:

- *What is it?*
  giving a brief summary of the current understanding of the nature of the condition.

- *Who gets it when?*
  showing the age-sex distributions and influence of other factors such as social class, international comparisons, and their likely frequency in general practice and at the district general hospital.

- *What happens?*
  analysing the significance of symptoms and signs, the likely course and outcome and how these influence care.

- *What to do?*
  an appreciation of the nature and presentation of the condition, and their relevance to diagnosis and management.

Our style and thinking have developed from experience with our previous books: *Common Diseases* (Fry, J., MTP, 1985), *Common Medical Problems* (Sandler, G., MTP, 1984) and *NHS Data Book* (Fry, J., Brooks, D., and McColl, I., MTP, 1984). As general practitioners and as a consultant physician in a district general hospital, we are aware of the real importance of being able to obtain a clear appreciation of our common problems in as easy and as quick a way as possible. Hence our rapid-read method, style and approach. We have enjoyed the challenge of putting the material together and we have all learnt much from each other. We hope that our readers too will enjoy and learn from our efforts.

To whom do we dedicate our book? We believe that all medical students, postgraduate trainees and clinicians will find it of value, as will our colleagues in associated para-medical professions.

John Fry
Gerald Sandler
David Brooks

Acknowledgements

G. S: I am greatly indebted to my secretary, Christine Green, who worked so indefatigably and efficiently in typing the manuscript. I would like to thank Philip Hickson and Neil Wimpenny for their help in the production of some of the illustrations. I would also like to thank sincerely my very understanding wife, Ella, who continues to have inexhaustible patience with my writing and with the inevitable neglect that it entails.

1   HIGH BLOOD PRESSURE

WHAT IS IT?

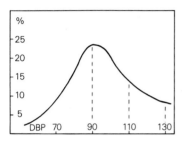

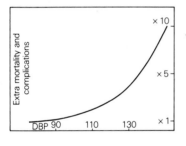

- high blood pressure' is unusual in that it is not a disease' *per se*. It is a diagnosis made by a machine, the sphygmomanometer, and it is made when the readings are above the arbitrary levels of 160/90

- blood pressures (both systolic and diastolic) have unimodal distributions in the population

- the importance of high blood pressure (systolic as well as diastolic) is that it becomes increasingly dangerous with complications as the pressures rise

- the risks of complications and death are directly related to the BP levels (systolic and diastolic)

- the levels of blood pressure in the population are related to

    age – rise with age

    sex – higher in females

    family traits – inherited tendency

    culture – higher in urbanized societies

    race – lower in Africans

    obesity – higher

    alcoholics – higher

    social class – 5 > 1

causes and types

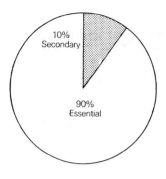

10%
Secondary

90%
Essential

- single definable causes of high blood pressure are uncommon
    - *secondary hypertension* makes up only 5–10% of cases (see pages 9 and 12 for causes)
- the great majority (90–95%) are '*essential hypertension*' (primary or of unknown cause)
- high blood pressure can be considered a variant of the normal and as a disease when it causes complications
- *complications*
    - strokes
    - heart failure
    - sudden heart attack (acute)
    - kidney damage
    - eye damage
- *malignant hypertension* (rare, less than 5% of all cases) with very high levels of blood pressure (> 250/140) and if untreated causes death usually within a year
- *some possible causes and mechanisms* which may be involved include
    - hormones such as noradrenaline, adrenaline, renin, angiotensin and related enzymes, aldosterone, prostaglandins and kinins
    - diet – salt (sodium) excess

Korotkow sounds

- the measurement of blood pressure by the sphygmomanometer depends on the *Korotkow sounds*

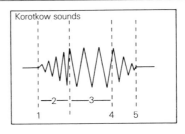

- Phase 1   Abrupt appearance of faint tapping sound
- Phase 2   Sounds prolonged into louder murmur
- Phase 3   Sounds clearer and more intense
- Phase 4   Sudden muffling of sounds
- Phase 5   Complete disappearance of sounds

There is still a controversy regarding whether the diastolic pressure should be the muffling of the sounds (phase 4) or the complete disappearance of the sounds (phase 5). In the UK phase 4 is most frequently used, and in the USA phase 5. Simultaneous comparison of the Korotkow sounds with direct intra-arterial pressure recording shows that phase 5 approximates better to the diastolic pressure than phase 4

WHO GETS IT AND WHEN?

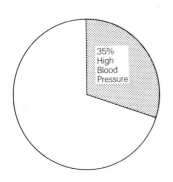

- at any time 10–15% of the population have high blood pressure (> 160/90) – this means 5–7 million in UK and 20–30 million in USA
- at least one third of middle-aged (over 40) and more of elderly will be hypertensive
- prevalence increases with age and is higher in females at all ages

frequency

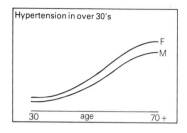

Hypertension in over 30's

F
M

30   age   70 +

- point prevalence of high blood pressure is up to 150 per 1000

- annual incidence (new cases) is likely to be five per 1000

general practice

hypertension in population of 2500

New cases diagnosed (annual incidence)	12
In practice (prevalence)	375
age 30–64	225
age 65+	150

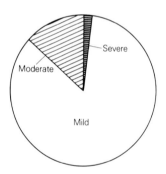

- *grades of severity of GP cases*

	Mild	Moderate	Severe	Total
DBP	(90–109)	(110–129)	(> 130)	
	320	50	5	375
	(85%)	(13.5%)	(1.5%)	(100)

district general hospital

DGH serving 250 000 (annual)

Referrals to OPD for difficulty in control of BP+	250
Admissions	
Hypertensive strokes	200
Hypertensive heart disease	100
Hypertensive other complications	50

WHAT HAPPENS?

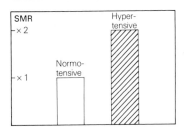

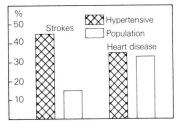

- high blood pressure doubles the risk of premature death (before age 70)
- majority of untreated hypertensives have normal life expectancies with no complications
- chief causes of death in hypertensives
  - strokes (45%)
  - heart disease (35%)
- death rates from *strokes* are 3 × those of the whole population
- deaths from *heart disease* proportionately not much greater than expected

risk factors

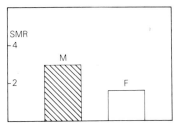

- *sex* – mortality risks are twice as high in males as females

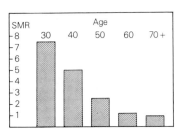

- *age at diagnosis*
  - inverse relationship of mortality rates and age at diagnosis
  - *note* over 60s have no appreciable extra mortality rates

- *family history* of deaths from strokes and high blood pressure increases mortality risk three-fold

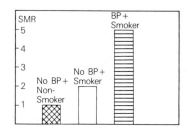

- *smoking* is added mortality risk factor

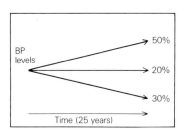

- BP levels do not inevitably rise with age. During 25 years of observation:

  50% went up

  20% stayed same

  30% went down

HOW DO THEY PRESENT?

symptoms

in the majority there are no symptoms that can be referred to the raised blood pressure

in 60% no symptoms

in 20% anxiety state

in 20% possible symptoms related to effects of raised blood pressure

hypertensive headache

the only symptom directly attributable to hypertension is headache. The typical features of the hypertensive headache are:

- level of blood pressure must be high diastolic pressure > 125 mm

- occipital

- throbbing

- on waking in the morning

- lasts several hours

most hypertensive patients who have headaches develop the headache after they learn that they are hypertensive. The distinctive features of this type of anxiety or 'tension' headache are:

- feeling of pressure, or tight band round the head, 'bursting', or other emotive and fanciful descriptions
- anywhere in the skull, often at vertex
- occurs any time, often at times of stress
- lasts seconds, hours, days, often 'all the time'

epistaxis   although this may be a presenting symptom in hypertension, it occurs frequently with normal blood pressure, owing to fragile blood vessels in Little's area in the nose

other symptoms   these may be related to atherosclerotic involvement of other organs consequent to the hypertension

- angina and breathlessness due to coronary artery disease
- dizziness due to cerebrovascular disease
- claudication due to peripheral vascular disease
- central abdominal pain and diarrhoea 15–30 min after a meal due to mesenteric artery disease
- visual deterioration due to retinal vascular disease
- polyuria, loss of weight, hiccoughs, twitching due to renal vascular disease and failure

signs
- in 70% no abnormal signs apart from raised blood pressure
- in 20% signs of cardiac strain
- in 10% signs of other organ damage
- signs of arteriosclerosis often present (Figure 1.1)

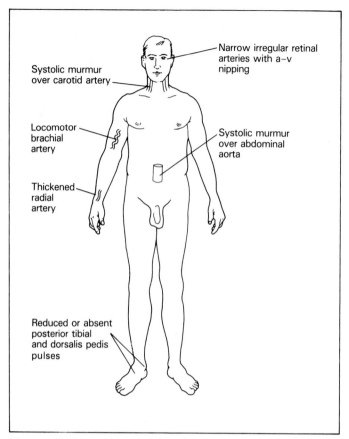

Figure 1.1 *Signs of arteriosclerosis*

level of blood pressure at diagnosis

- mild (90–109 mm DBP) 85%
- moderate (110 – 129 mm DBP) 13.5%
- severe (above 130 mm DBP) 1.5%

cardiac strain

high blood pressure is the commonest cause of left ventricular failure. The signs which indicate this are

- breathlessness
- gallop rhythm
- showers of fine crepitations in the lungs, especially at the bases

secondary hypertension

90–95% of patients who present with hypertension have essential hypertension. The most useful diagnostic clue is a family history of hypertension: if both parents are hypertensive, half the offspring may be hypertensive – if only one parent, the risk falls to 25%. Some diagnostic help in the 5–10% of patients whose hypertension is secondary, most of whom are in the younger age groups, may be provided by the history and the clinical examination. Relevant features in the history are

- past history of kidney disease
- family history of 'Bright's disease' or polycystic kidney
- present history

    frequency, dysuria, loin pain → kidney disease
    attacks of headache, sweating, trembling → phaeochromocytoma

    severe weakness and polyuria → Conn's syndrome

    constitutional symptoms, muscle and joint pain, pleurisy, pericardiac pain, abdominal pain, asthma, paraesthesiae → polyarteritis nodosa

- drugs

    'the pill'

    alcohol

    steroids

signs

the *signs* which may be helpful in the diagnosis of secondary hypertension are shown in Figure 1.2

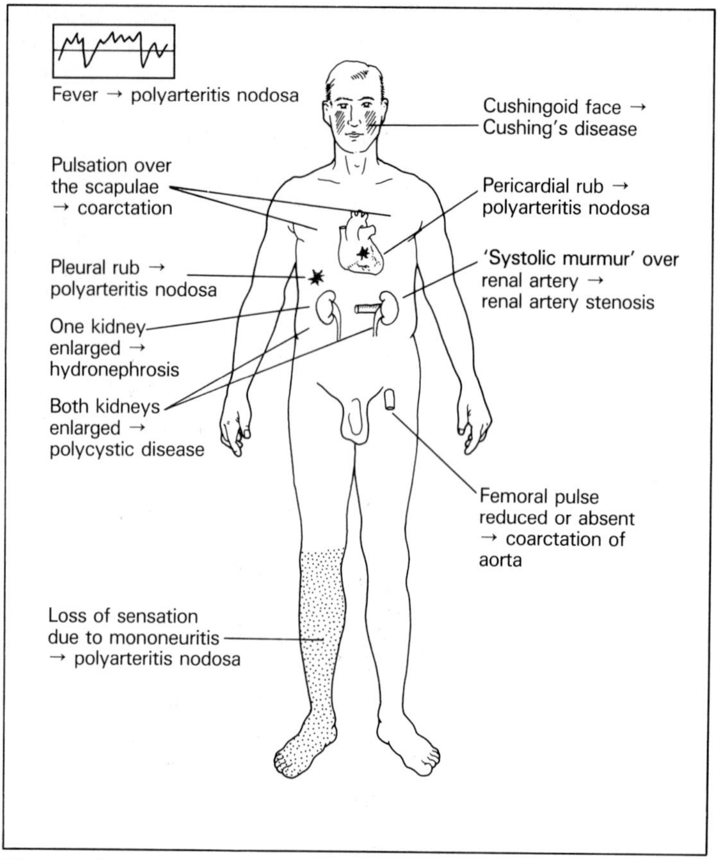
Fever → polyarteritis nodosa
Cushingoid face → Cushing's disease
Pulsation over the scapulae → coarctation
Pericardial rub → polyarteritis nodosa
Pleural rub → polyarteritis nodosa
'Systolic murmur' over renal artery → renal artery stenosis
One kidney enlarged → hydronephrosis
Both kidneys enlarged → polycystic disease
Femoral pulse reduced or absent → coarctation of aorta
Loss of sensation due to mononeuritis → polyarteritis nodosa

Figure 1.2 *Signs in secondary hypertension*

WHAT TO DO?

there is no one specific management that can confidently be expected to be completely successful because of the uncertainties of causes and unpredictability of the natural history in mild–moderate grades

steps in assessment

is there a *raised BP* – based on readings on at least three separate occasions?

what *risk factors* are present?

- age – younger patients have worse prognosis
- sex – males have worse prognosis
- family history of premature death from hypertension, coronary disease or

cerebrovascular disease implies a worse prognosis

- blood pressure level – systolic and diastolic – related directly to prognosis
- smoking greatly enhances the risk of developing a serious vascular complication
- high cholesterol level carries a worse prognosis, but probably worth checking only in younger patients (< 40 years)
- diabetes worsens prognosis
- obesity worsens prognosis but only slightly
- contraceptive pill in hypertensive women may lead to a heart attack or stroke, especially if the woman is also a smoker

check

The signs to look for are shown in Figure 1.3

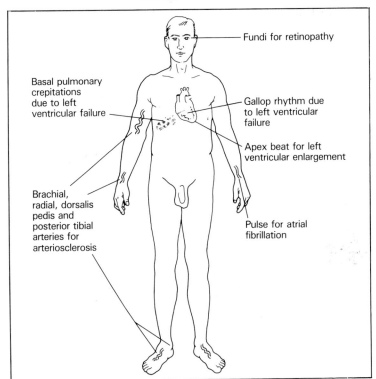

Basal pulmonary crepitations due to left ventricular failure

Fundi for retinopathy

Gallop rhythm due to left ventricular failure

Apex beat for left ventricular enlargement

Brachial, radial, dorsalis pedis and posterior tibial arteries for arteriosclerosis

Pulse for atrial fibrillation

Figure 1.3   *Signs in hypertension*

investigations

essential hypertension

the purpose of investigation in essential hypertension is to help in deciding prognosis

- urine – proteinuria suggests worse prognosis – haematuria suggests malignant hypertension
- chest X-ray – for cardiac enlargement – poorer prognosis
- e.c.g. – for left ventricular hypertrophy ± strain – adverse prognosis
- e.c.g. – for ischaemic changes – indicates associated coronary disease
- blood urea – for renal failure
- serum creatinine – more sensitive than blood urea in picking up early renal failure

secondary hypertension

the tests which may be of value in detecting secondary hypertension are

- serum K – low in hyperaldosteronism (Conn's syndrome)
- chest X-ray – notched ribs in coarctation
- i.v.p. – unilateral or bilateral renal disease
- renal arteriogram for renal artery stenosis
- urinary VMA excretion – for pheochromocytoma
- blood cortisol level – for Cushing's syndrome

MANAGEMENT

unless regular (3–5-yearly) blood pressure measurements are taken on all adults who consult, real and potential hypertensives will not be diagnosed and preventive opportunities missed. It is only after a persistent (on three separate occasions at a week or more interval) raised level of blood pressure is found (> 160/90) that decisions on treatment can be taken

The questions which the doctor has to answer when faced with a hypertensive patient are

- who to treat?
- who not to treat?
- what drugs to use and in what order?

which patients should be treated right away

the hypertensive patients requiring *urgent treatment* are

- malignant hypertension

    severe blood pressure 250+/140+

    grade 4 retinopathy

    uraemia

- target organ damage

    heart – angina, left ventricular failure

    brain – haemorrhage, stroke

    kidneys – renal failure

- level of blood pressure

    systolic > 220 mm

    diastolic > 110 mm

with lesser degrees of blood pressure (diastolic 95–110 mm) the factors which suggest treatment are

- young patient < 50 years
- male patient
- bad family history
- other adverse prognostic factors

    high cholesterol

    intractable cigarette smoking

    diabetes

which patients should probably not be treated

- labile hypertension – just observe
- > 60 years

- females with mild hypertension

    systolic < 220 mm

    diastolic < 110 mm

- obesity – try weight reduction first
- smokers who are able to give up – assess effects on blood pressure first
- no adverse family history and no other adverse prognostic factors

what treatment should be given

general measures

- control of risk factors

    smoking

    high cholesterol (in young patients < 40 years)

    treat diabetes

    stop contraceptive pill

- reduce weight if obese
- reduce salt intake – no added salt
- reduce intake of alcohol
- recheck blood pressure regularly

specific treatment

which drugs should be given and in what order? The basic groups of hypertensive drugs are

- diuretics
- β-blockers
- peripheral vasodilators

diuretics

- a thiazide diuretic could be the first line of treatment (especially in elderly). The drugs in common use are

    hydrochlorothiazide (Hydrosaluric): 25–100 mg daily

    bendrofluazide (Aprinox): 2.5–5.0 mg daily

cyclopenthiazide (Navidrex):
0.25–0.5 mg daily

- the side-effects of thiazides are

    hyperglycaemia → exacerbation of
    diabetes

    hypokalaemia → fatigue

    hyperuricaemia → gout

    impotence in young males

- if hypokalaemia develops, a potassium-
  sparing diuretic can be substituted or added

    triamterene (Dytac)
    150–250 mg daily

    amiloride (Midamor)
    5–10 mg daily

    spironolactone (Aldactone)
    50–100 mg daily

β-blockers

these drugs may be used as first-line treatment
(especially in young) or added to the thiazide if
blood pressure control is inadequate. The
β-blocking drugs currently available are
shown in Table 1.1

Table 1.1   *Selectivity and dose of β-blockers*

Drug	Selectivity	Daily dose (mg)
Acebutolol (Sectral)	cardioselective	400–1200
Atenolol (Tenormin)	cardioselective	50–100
Metoprolol (Betaloc)	cardioselective	100–400
Nadolol (Corgard)	non-selective	80–240
Oxprenolol (Trasicor)	non-selective	120–480
Propranolol (Inderal)	non-selective	160–320
Sotalol (Sotacor)	non-selective	80–600
Timolol (Prestim)	non-selective	10–60

the side-effects of the β-blockers are

- bronchospasm

- precipitation left ventricular failure

- claudication

- fatigue
- impotence
- masking of hypoglycaemia
- nightmares and hallucinations

peripheral vasodilators

- these drugs are third-line treatment. The drugs in current use are

    hydralazine

    prazosin

    minoxidil

- *hydralazine* is the most effective drug

    direct vasodilator

    25 mg t.d.s. – 50 mg q.d.s.

    side-effects – postural dizziness
    flushing
    throbbing headache
    ankle swelling
    'SLE'

    combine with a β-blocker to prevent reflex tachycardia

- *minoxidil* is reserved for resistant hypertension

    powerful direct vasodilator

    5 – 50 mg daily in divided doses

    side-effects – weight gain
    oedema
    hirsutes
    gastrointestinal upset
    tender breasts

other

- methyldopa (Aldomet) still remains a useful drug

    action – central on brain
    peripheral on sympathetic
    nerves

    250 mg t.d.s. – 500 mg q.d.s.

                    side-effects – drowsiness
                                   depression
                                   fatigue
                                   diarrhoea
                                   impotence

                    rare toxicity – parkinsonism
                                    chronic hepatitis
                                    haemolytic anaemia

resistant hypertension   a minority of hypertensive patients will be
                                     resistant to all the previous treatment. It may
                                     be desirable to have specialist advice for these
                                     patients. The approach to management of
                                     these patients is

- check patient is taking his drugs

- ensure maximal doses of drugs have been
  tried

- use a loop diuretic (Lasix, Burinex) to
  counteract fluid retention

- exclude neutralizing actions of any drugs
  given concurrently

      tricyclic antidepressants
      adrenal steroids
      oestrogens

   try other hypotensive drugs

      calcium-antagonist (Adalat)
      labetalol – α- and β-blocker
      captopril – angiotensin-converting-
      enzyme inhibitor (Capoten)
      enalapril (Innovace)

what benefits to be expected with treatment

                    the likely benefits are:

- reduced mortality

      certainly in young severe hypertensives
      who smoke

      less certainly in older patients and in fat
      women in whom prognosis is favourable
      anyway

- reduced chance of heart failure
- reduced chance of a haemorrhagic stroke
- reduced chance of hypertensive renal failure
- likely reduction in incidence of heart attacks

well-being

- even well-controlled hypertensive patients are unlikely to feel better
- the side-effects of the drugs used may well make the patient feel worse, especially β-blockers which frequently cause fatigue and lack of drive
- the angiotensin-converting-enzyme inhibitors are claimed to produce a feeling of well-being, quite unlike most other antihypertensive drugs

  captopril (Capoten)

  enalapril (Innovace)

efficacy of control

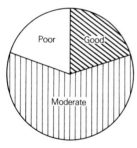

it must not be assumed that control of raised blood pressure is easily achieved

in spite of use of the large range of drugs by GPs and specialists the results are not that good

- *good* control (DBP < 90 mm) in 20%
- *moderate* control (DBP 90 – 109 mm) in 60%
- *poor* control (DBP > 110 mm) in 20%

Useful practical points

- high blood pressure cannot be readily accepted as a 'disease' affecting around one third of all adults particularly as we are unclear of its nature, causes and outcome
- most are of mild–moderate grades and many are elderly with good prognosis
- great majority (90%) are 'essential' or of unknown cause
- for all these reasons management has to be tentative and pragmatic
- high blood pressure does carry extra risks of stroke death particularly in men under 65
- all adults should have their blood pressures recorded every 3–5 years
- all confirmed (at least three raised BP readings) hypertensives should be under regular supervision and those under 60–65 actively managed
- indications for urgent treatment:

    BP + + (> 220/110)

    target organ damage

    young (< 50 years)

    males

    bad F.H.
- before embarking on drug treatment, time should be given for non-medication measures to lower BP such as

    weight reduction

    mental/physical relaxation

    no smoking

    reduction of salt intake

    reduction of alcohol
- step-by-step therapeutic scheme

    diuretic

    β-blocker

    vasodilator   -

    other
- however, even with intensive drug therapy good control may not be achieved

2 ISCHAEMIC HEART DISEASE

WHAT IS IT?

- ischaemic heart disease (IHD) is a collective term for a local cardiac manifestation of a generalized body disorder, arteriosclerosis (Figure 2.1)

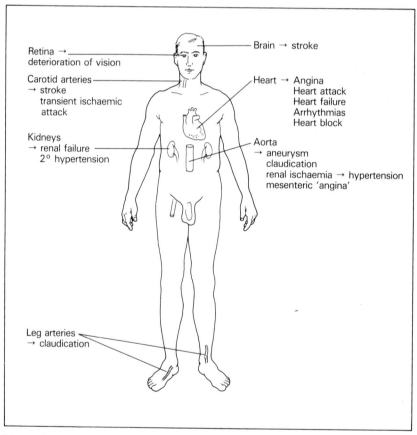

Figure 2.1 *Generalized arteriosclerosis and its clinical manifestations*

- atheroma affects the three main coronary arteries (see Figure 2.2)

  left circumflex

  anterior descending

  right coronary artery

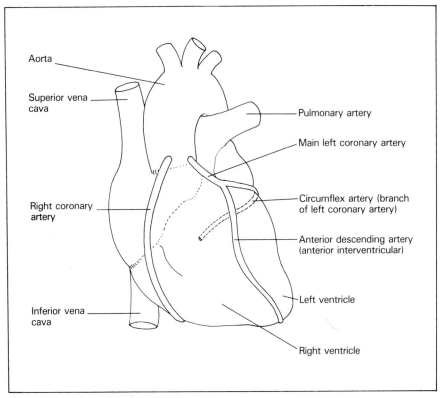

Figure 2.2   *Coronary artery anatomy*

- there is poor correlation between the morbid anatomy of the coronary arteries at autopsy and the clinical course during life
- there is a better correlation between coronary artery anatomy seen on angiography during life and the clinical manifestations

clinical presentation

- *angina* – ischaemia of myocardium – when the demand for blood outstrips the supply through the narrowed coronary arteries

- *myocardial infarction*: – complete and sustained cut-off of blood supply to myocardium leading to necrosis of muscle
- *sudden death*: – sudden, unheralded and unexpected – in most cases due to 'electrocution' of the heart from ventricular fibrillation
- *other clinical manifestations* of coronary artery disease

    left ventricular failure

    cardiac arrhythmias

    heart block (Stokes–Adams attacks)

    emboli from silent myocardial infarction

    > brain → stroke

    > limbs → gangrene

risk factors

No single cause of IHD but risk factors can be defined

major
- cigarette smoking
- hypertension
- hypercholesterolaemia

minor
- family history

    premature coronary disease

    premature arterial disease

    hypertension
- diabetes
- obesity
- contraceptive pill (especially smokers)
- premature menopause
- 'soft water'

dubious
- psychological stress
- sedentary life with little exercise

WHO GETS IT AND WHEN?

difficult to determine exact incidence and prevalence rates of mortality and morbidity

coronary arteriosclerosis is almost universal in adults of developed countries

exact diagnosis may be difficult and imprecise even at autopsy or with intensive investigations

rates will vary whether they come from population screening, hospitals, general practice or autopsy

clinical presentations

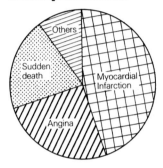

- sudden death (20%)
- myocardial infarction (45%)
- angina (25%)
- others (10%)

age and sex incidence

- IHD is a disease of ageing
- more frequent in males at younger ages, with females 'catching up' after 60

frequency

general practice

annual incidence (new cases) in population of 2500

Sudden deaths from IHD	3
Acute myocardial infarction	7
Angina	4
Others	1
	15

(note that in this population there will be seven to eight deaths from IHD in a year – this includes the three sudden deaths) annual prevalence (patients consulting) of all forms of IHD

Myocardial infarction and after	15
Angina	25
Heart failure	25
Others	5
	70

district general hospital (DGH)

- in 1982 there were 150 090 deaths and discharges from IHD in NHS hospitals in England and Wales[2]
- of these approximately 30 000 were deaths
- an average DGH will admit 600 IHD cases a year and of those about 100 will die in hospital

DGH serving 250 000

Admissions	
acute myocardial infarction	500
(deaths in hospital)	(100)
heart failure and other reasons	100

WHAT HAPPENS?

mortality

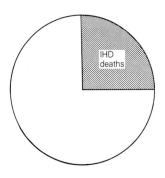

- IHD is the largest single cause of death in developed countries (a quarter of all deaths). In 1975 in England and Wales

    deaths from IHD: *154 371*

    total deaths: *583 000*

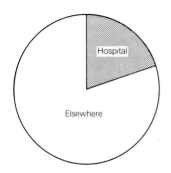

- only 20% (30 000) of IHD deaths take place in hospital, others (80%) at home and elsewhere (street, work etc)

- IHD mortality increases with age, but one quarter of all IHD deaths are in persons under 65

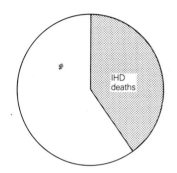

- IHD is a major cause of premature death in males more than females. In males aged 45–60, 40% of all deaths are from IHD

mortality trends

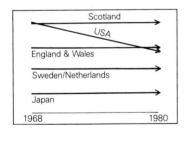

- since 1968 IHD mortality rates have been falling in USA and Australia, but have remained static in Scotland, England and Wales, Netherlands, Sweden and Japan (Rose 1981). It is likely that UK rates have begun to decline in 1980s[9]

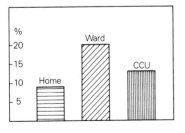

- *acute myocardial infarction*: mortality rates by place of treatment[10]

    Home 9% (selected)

    Ward 20%

    Coronary care unit 13%

outcomes (5-year follow-up)

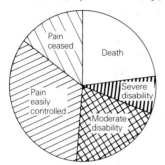

- *angina*

    14% pain ceased or insignificant

    35% easily controlled with medication

    20% moderate disability

    8% severe disability (candidates for surgery)

    23% deaths

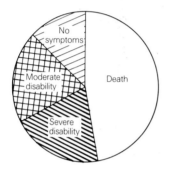

- *myocardial infarction* (5-year follow-up)

    13% no symptoms

    20% moderate disability

    20% severe disability

    47% deaths

IHD deaths

early deaths (first month)

- 30% of all IHD deaths occur *within 4 weeks* of clinical diagnosis

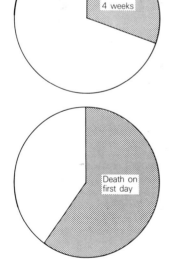

- 60% of all early (first month) deaths occur on *first day*

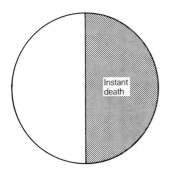

- 50% of all first day deaths occur *within 15 minutes* (instant deaths)

WHAT TO DO?

- IHD is a modern epidemic
- IHD is not a single clinical disorder, e.g. angina, myocardial infarction, heart failure, arrhythmias
- IHD is more of a 'social' disease due to personal factors
- IHD is preventable (to a degree)

issues

- *issue* – how much preventable? Falling US mortality trends suggest it is feasible though with all the multifactorial measures employed it is still not clear whether the fall is due to intervention or some other unknown factor
- *issue* – should prevention be responsibility of individual, doctor or community?
- *issue* – how realistic is it to tackle preventable causes, i.e.

  hypertension?

  smoking?

  hypercholesterolaemia?

- *issue* – medical treatment is largely

  a 'band-aid' exercise in managing *effects* of IHD

  acute attacks: 'keep alive' home or hospital?

  ward or CCU?

  long term care: medication

  other measures

  diet

         lifestyle

         exercise

- *issue* – surgery is largely a 'plumbing' exercise to bypass obstructed coronary arteries and increase the blood supply to ischaemic myocardium

    who are candidates?

    when should surgery be considered?

    what are the benefits?

    what are the risks?

diagnosis of ischaemic heart disease

angina

history

the diagnosis of angina is made principally on the history; investigations have very little contribution to make in deciding whether a patient's chest pain is due to angina

the diagnosis is based on the characteristics of the chest pain

- site
- radiation
- character
- duration
- precipitating factors
- relieving factors
- associated symptoms
- *site of pain*

    classically behind sternum

    sometimes left chest

    rarely right chest

    very rarely back

- *radiation* (Figure 2.3)

    left arm commonest

    right arm sometimes

    both arms sometimes

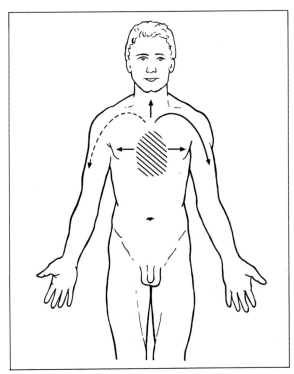

Figure 2.3 *Radiation of angina*

throat

chin

back of neck – occasional

epigastrium – rare

through to back – rare

sometimes pain reverses – starts in left wrist or arm and radiates back to chest

sometimes pain in left arm without chest pain

- *character of pain*

  very suggestive   gripping

  squeezing

  crushing

  constricting

  'like a vice'

  'like a tight band'

less convincing	ache
	pressure
	cramping
	heaviness
arm pain	lifelessness
	deadness
	uselessness
	tingling – much more dubious

- *duration of pain*

  angina lasts 5 – 10 min once the causative factor has been removed

  it never lasts for a few seconds only

  it never lasts for hours – if it does consider

coronary spasm	Prinzmetal's angina
	rest angina
	unstable angina

  myocardial infarction

- *precipitating factors*

  exertion – most important factor

  mental stress, emotion

  cold wind

  heavy meal

- *relieving factors*

  stopping exertion

  glyceryl trinitrate – response should occur in 1–2 min

- *associated symptoms*

  'choking' in the throat – highly suggestive of angina

  'strangling' and 'suffocation' also highly suggestive

  breathlessness – transient left ventricular failure

  dizziness – could be anxiety

  syncope – rare

belching at end of attack

examination in angina

- there may be no abnormal physical signs at all
- there may be signs of arteriosclerosis (Figure 2.4)

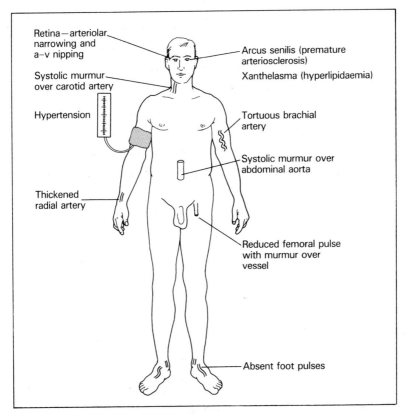

Retina — arteriolar narrowing and a–v nipping

Systolic murmur over carotid artery

Hypertension

Thickened radial artery

Arcus senilis (premature arteriosclerosis)

Xanthelasma (hyperlipidaemia)

Tortuous brachial artery

Systolic murmur over abdominal aorta

Reduced femoral pulse with murmur over vessel

Absent foot pulses

Figure 2.4   *Signs of arteriosclerosis*

- hypertension is often present
- there may be signs of hyperlipidaemia

  xanthelasma

  arcus senilis

  xanthomata

  tendons

  skin – extensor surfaces

differential diagnosis of angina

- *functional pain*

    left mammary or inframammary

    stabbing or continuous ache

    lasts seconds, hours, days

    unrelated to exertion

    often while relaxing and introspective

    other anxiety symptoms

    local tenderness in chest wall

- *pleuritic pain*

    localized to one side

    sharp, stabbing, knife-like

    worse with inspiration, coughing

    associated phlegm   purulent (infection)

    blood (embolism)

    pleural rub on auscultation

- *hiatus hernia*

    retrosternal burning pain

    worse   on bending

    on lying in bed

    after heavy meal

    associated with heartburn

- *peptic ulcer*

    epigastric and lower sternal pain

    deep gnawing pain

    related to meals

    relieved by alkalis

    may be associated with vomiting which relieves the pain

    epigastric tenderness

- *pericarditis*

    retrosternal pain

    worse on lying, better on standing, sitting up

worse with inspiration, cough

may hear pericardial rub

- *cervical spondylosis*

  upper chest pain

  involves shoulders and arms

  unrelated to exertion

  worse with movements of neck

  often crepitus on moving head

investigation of angina

- *electrocardiogram*

  this is of very little value in the diagnosis of angina since it is often normal

  if recorded during an actual angina attack it may show S–T depression (Figure 2.5)

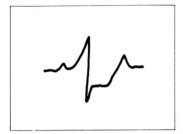

Figure 2.5   *e.c.g. – ST ↓ in angina*

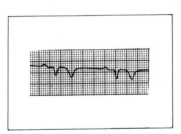

Figure 2.6   *e.c.g. – old infarction*

it may show evidence of previous myocardial infarction (Figure 2.6)

exercise e.c.g. may be of more value in showing ST depression during exercise. However, this will only help in the diagnosis of the chest pain if the actual pain occurs during exercise and is correlated with ischaemic S–T depression in the e.c.g. trace (Figure 2.7)

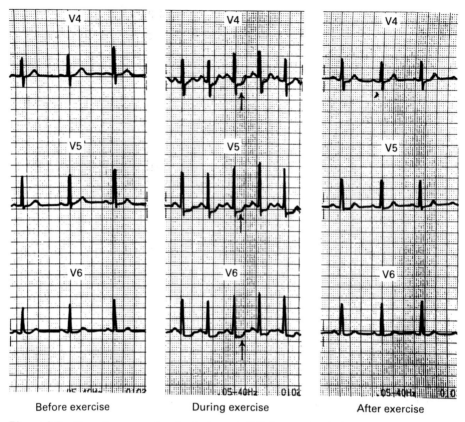

| Before exercise | During exercise | After exercise |

Figure 2.7 *Exercise e.c.g. showing ischaemic S-T depression during exercise*

- *arteriography* – coronary arteriography is the definitive test in diagnosing coronary artery disease
- *thallium studies* – radionuclide studies with radioactive thallium are also of value in showing ischaemic areas developing in the myocardium after exercise ('cold spots')

diagnosis of myocardial infarction

> *history*

- *pain* – the site, character and radiation of the pain are identical with those of angina pectoris – the distinguishing features are pain much more severe

more prolonged – over half an hour and
often several hours

often occurs at rest, especially in bed

no relief with glyceryl trinitrate

● *associated symptoms*

breathlessness often due to left
ventricular failure

sweating and nausea/vomiting are almost
invariable

dizziness due to lowered cardiac output

syncope more likely than in angina

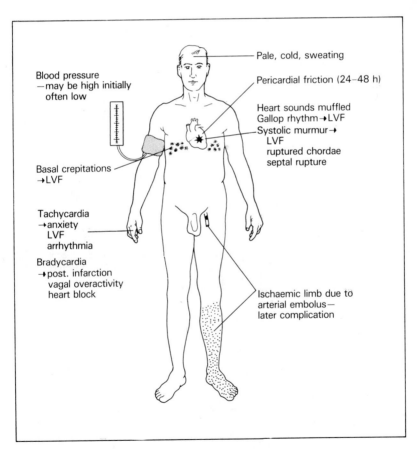

Blood pressure
—may be high initially
often low

Pale, cold, sweating

Pericardial friction (24–48 h)

Heart sounds muffled
Gallop rhythm→LVF
Systolic murmur→
LVF
ruptured chordae
septal rupture

Basal crepitations
→LVF

Tachycardia
→anxiety
LVF
arrhythmia

Bradycardia
→post. infarction
vagal overactivity
heart block

Ischaemic limb due to
arterial embolus—
later complication

Figure 2.8 *Possible signs in myocardial infarction*

palpitations often due to cardiac arrhythmias

fear of impending death (angor animi)

examination

- like angina there may be no abnormal signs

- the possible findings are shown in Figure 2.8

investigations

- *electrocardiogram*

    this is the most important test and is mandatory in all suspected cases

    the changes are shown in Figure 2.9

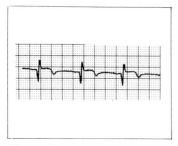

Figure 2.9 *e.c.g. changes in myocardial infarction*

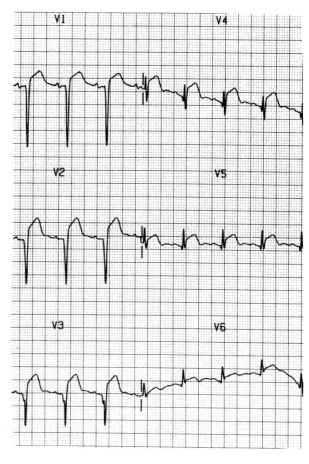

Figure 2.10 *e.c.g. showing changes of acute anterior infarction in the anterior chest leads*

ISCHAEMIC HEART DISEASE

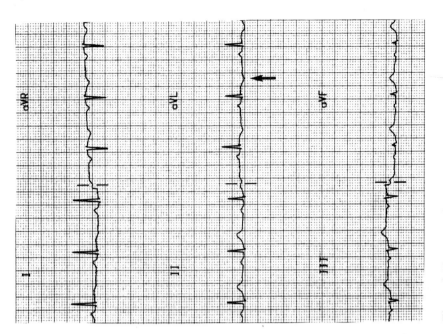
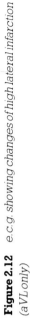

Figure 2.12 *e.c.g. showing changes of high lateral infarction (aVL only)*

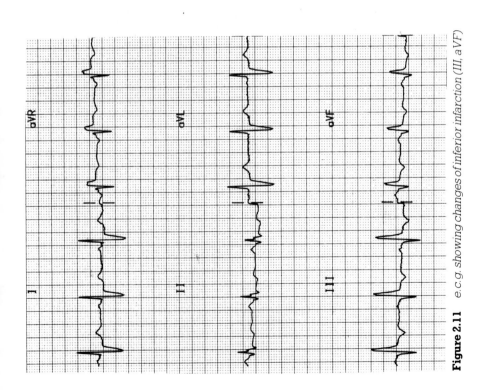

Figure 2.11 *e.c.g. showing changes of inferior infarction (III, aVF)*

Q waves – myocardial necrosis

ST elevation – myocardial injury

T inversion – myocardial ischaemia

the site of the infarction is indicated by the
e.c.g. leads affected

anterior – I aVL V1–V6 (Figure 2.10)

posterior – III

inferior III – aVF (Figure 2.11)

high lateral – aVL (Figure 2.12)

persistent S–T elevation suggests the
possibility of ventricular aneurysm

Q waves indicative of myocardial necrosis
are usually permanent

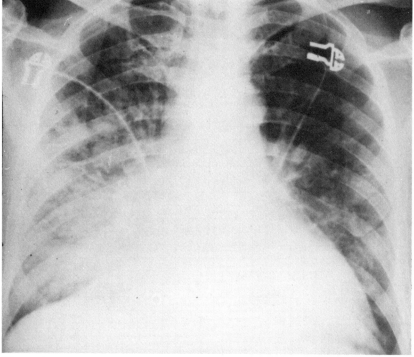

Figure 2.13   *Chest X-ray showing pulmonary oedema especially in the right lung*

- *cardiac enzymes*

    these are enzymes released into the
    circulation from damaged myocardial
    cells

ISCHAEMIC HEART DISEASE

they are very helpful in

diagnosis of infarction

prognosis – the higher the level of serum enzymes the worse the prognosis

they are released into the blood at different time intervals after the infarction

Enzyme*	Starts	Peaks	Ends
CPK	4–6 h	12 h	72 h
AST	12 h	1–2 days	5 days
LDH	12 h	2–3 days	7 days

* CPK – creatinine phosphokinase; AST – aspartate aminotransferase (formerly glutamic oxaloacetic transaminase – SGOT); LDH – lactic dehydrogenase

false positive increases of cardiac enzymes may occur after

intramuscular injections

left ventricular failure

pulmonary embolism

muscle disease

red cell damage

to overcome these false positive results the enzyme measurements can be refined to identify the cardiac component of the enzymes

CPK → CPK-MB

LDH → LDH$_1$

- *chest X-ray*: the relevant findings in myocardial infarction are

LV failure

congested upper lobe veins

basal congestion

pulmonary oedema with hilar flare (Figure 2.13)

cardiac enlargement – bad prognostic sign

- *other blood tests*

  leukocytosis – non-specific – very little diagnostic help

  ESR ↑ – non-specific

  blood sugar ↑ – myocardial infarction may show up latent diabetes

TREATMENT

angina

aims

- to relieve symptoms
- to improve function
- to prevent complications

  myocardial infarction

  cardiac arrhythmia

  sudden death
- to prolong life

general

- stop cigarette smoking
- control high blood pressure
- reduce obesity
- correct anaemia
- alter lifestyle if possible

  cut working week

  regular holidays

  adequate and enjoyable leisure

  regular exercise

  avoid emotional crises work/home if possible
- reduce hypercholesterolaemia – mainly benefits younger patient (< 40 years)

  diet
  cholestyramine (Questran)

specific

- *nitrates*

    mainstay of treatment

    use sublingual glyceryl trinitrate

    - to relieve pain

    - to prevent pain

    sorbide mononitrate (Monit, Elantan) 10–30 mg up to q.d.s. for prophylaxis

    percutaneous (Transiderm-Nitro 5 mg, 10 mg)

    - daily for prophylaxis but probably effective only for first few hours after application

    - can be used for nocturnal angina

- *β-blockers*

    often very effective (except where angina is due primarily to coronary spasm)

    drugs available

    - propranolol (Inderal) 120–360 mg/day

    - atenolol (Tenormin) 100–200 mg/day

    - metoprolol (Betaloc) 100–200 mg/day

    - oxprenolol (Trasicor) 120–480 mg/day

    - acebutolol (Sectral) 300–800 mg/day

    - timolol (Betim) 15–45 mg/day

    - sotalol (Sotacor) 160–480 mg/day

    - nadolol (Corgard) 40–240 mg/day

    - pindolol (Visken) 7.5–45 mg/day

    all equally effective in angina

    cardioselective best (atenolol, metoprolol, acebutolol) in some cases:

    - associated bronchospasm in chronic lung disease

    - intermittent claudication

    - diabetes

    side-effects

    - bronchospasm

precipitation of latent heart failure

peripheral vasoconstriction

  cold extremities

  claudication

fatigue – frequent

impotence

masking of hypoglycaemia in diabetes

nightmares, insomnia (propranolol)

- *calcium antagonists*

valuable in angina especially when due to coronary spasm – Prinzmetal's angina

        rest angina

        unstable angina

nifedipine best (Adalat); 10–20 mg t.d.s.

side-effects

  postural dizziness

  flushing

  oedema

  GI upset

surgery for angina

- indications

intractable after full medical treatment with

  nitrates

  β-blocker

  Ca-antagonist

left main stem or anterior descending artery obstruction, especially in younger patient

multivessel disease – prognosis probably better with surgery

- types of surgery

angioplasty – for single vessel disease

bypass with vein grafts – up to six possible

- benefits of surgery (bypass operation)

80% of patients lose angina in 1st year

50% free of angina after 5 years

still controversial about prolongation of life in multivessel disease

- mortality of bypass operation = 1–2%

myocardial infarction

general treatment

- relief of pain – diamorphine
- allay anxiety

  verbal reassurance

  tranquillizer
- oxygen – probably worthwhile in all patients
- correct hypokalaemia – predisposes to arrhythmias
- careful observation with e.c.g. monitoring for first few hours because of risks of catastrophic arrhythmias

specific treatment

this is the treatment of the complications

- *LV failure*

  diuretics

  oxygen if not already given

  vasodilators if severe

  i.v. nitroprusside

  oral captopril 12.5 mg t.d.s. or enalapril 10 mg/day

- *arrhythmias*

  bradyarrhythmias

  tachyarrhythmias

  bradyarrythmias

  sinus bradycardia – especially with inferior infarction – treat if

  reduced cardiac output, e.g. low BP, dizziness

  ventricular ectopic beats

  treat –

  atropine s.c. or i.m.

temporary pacing if necessary

heart block – treat

2° Mobitz (dropped beats)

complete

bundle-branch block with abnormal axis

use temporary pacing wire

permanent implanted pacemaker if it doesn't clear up

tachyarrythmias

treat

frequent unifocal ventricular ectopics

ventricular ectopics in salvos

multifocal ectopics

R-on-T ectopics – *very* hazardous → ventricular fibrillation

ventricular tachycardia

many antiarrhythmic drugs available

i.v. lignocaine infusion best for ventricular arrhythmias

verapamil
disopyramide } for atrial arrhythmias

disopyramide
tocainide } for ventricular arrhythmias
flecainide

amiodarone for resistant supraventricular and ventricular arrhythmias

- *cardiogenic shock* – very bad prognosis – 90–95% mortality

inotropic agent – dobutamine, dopamine

vasodilators – i.v. nitroprusside

large doses steroids, e.g. Solumedrone 1 g i.m. 6-hrly

intraaortic balloon pump if available
N.B. All patients should have haemodynamic
monitoring to record pulmonary wedge pressure
(indirect left atrial pressure) and cardiac output

- *ventricular aneurysm*

    persistent S-T elevation in e.c.g.

    bulging left cardiac border on X-ray

    angiocardiography confirms

    treat – resection

- *other complications*

    ruptured chordae tendinae

    sudden LV failure

    mitral incompetence on examination

    treat – urgent surgery

    ruptured interventricular septum

    similar findings to ruptured chordae

    treat – urgent surgery if LV failure

PROGNOSIS

angina

- stable angina – annual mortality 4% (cf healthy men 45–54 → 0.9%)
- unstable angina – mortality in 1st year 17%
- prognosis depends on extent and location of coronary artery involvement

    one vessel : 1–2% per year

    two vessels 6% per year

    three vessels : 10% per year

    left main stem disease : 20% per year

- left ventricular failure greatly worsens the prognosis – 80% mortality within 5 years

myocardial infarction

- hospital mortality

    ward 20%

    CCU 13%

half the deaths < 2 h

75% of deaths < 24 h

30–40% deaths < 1/12

- long term

    > 80% live at least 1 year

    75% live for 5 years

    50% live for 10 years

    25% live for 15 years

PREVENTION OF IHD

- primary prevention is much more likely to be effective than secondary prevention – it is never too early to start and the most fruitful approach is likely to be with children

- the most important prophylactic measure of all is to prevent cigarette smoking

- other coronary risk factors are capable of modifications but the benefits are either limited or unproven

    control of hypertension – even mild

    reduction of cholesterol – more likely to be efficacious in young people

    reduction of obesity – limited value

    encourage regular exercise – dubious value

    avoid contraceptive pill especially in older woman who is a smoker

- with regard to secondary prophylaxis, the most useful drug is a β-blocker for which there is now ample and convincing evidence of value: the recommended drugs are timolol (Betim) or propranolol (Inderal). The drug can be started about a week after the heart attack and is effective for 3 years – what happens after that time is not yet known

thrombolysis

- this is a newer method of treatment which is currently being evaluated in the treatment of *early* myocardial infarction (< 3 h of onset). It involves using streptokinase to dissolve the thrombus in the coronary artery. It is administered in two ways:

direct intracoronary – through an intra-arterial catheter – requires special facilities

intravenous infusion – almost as effective – more suitable for general use

- the place of thrombolysis in the routine management of myocardial infarction remains to be established

home versus hospital treatment

the factors which help to decide whether a heart attack patient should be treated in hospital rather than at home:

- time factor – within few hours of onset
- complications

  heart failure

  cardiac arrhythmias

  shock (though resuscitate before)

  heartblock
- young patient (older may do better at home)
- patient's preference
- unsatisfactory home environment and help
- presence of a coronary care unit in the hospital
- availability of a coronary ambulance for potentially hazardous ambulance journey in a complicated patient

Useful practical points

- don't forget that anxious patients with functional pain can also develop angina

- belching after an attack of chest pain does not necessarily mean that the pain is gastro-oesophageal – belching may occur at the end of an authentic attack of angina

- don't consider that angina has failed medical treatment until the patient has had nitrates, a β-blocker and a Ca-antagonist

- control of hypercholesterolaemia is unlikely to have any significant clinical benefits in a middle-aged patient: it is of more value long-term in the young

- giving up cigarette smoking is the greatest single preventive public-health measure to reduce the incidence of coronary artery disease

3   STROKES

WHAT ARE THEY?

features

- sudden onset
- clinical signs of focal/global disturbance of cerebral function
- persist for more than 24 hours
- *note*: 'transient ischaemic attacks' – *TIA* – last for *less* than 24 h
- caused by vascular disorder
- *note*: excluded are other causes such as epilepsy, neoplasms, migraine and subdural and extradural haematomas

types

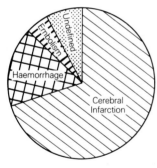

- cerebral infarction (70%)
- cerebral haemorrhage (17%)
- cerebral embolism (5%)
- others : undefined (8%)

cerebral infarction

- *commonest cause* is atheroma of cerebral arteries
- *other causes*
  - arteritis
    - polyarteritis nodosa
    - systemic lupus erythematosus

      giant cell (temporal arteritis)

      scleroderma (rare)

      rheumatoid arthritis

   blood

      polycythaemia (1° and 2°)

      essential thrombocythaemia

      myeloma (hyperviscosity)

      sickle-cell disease

   oral contraceptives

cerebral haemorrhage

causes

- hypertension → microaneurysms (Charcot–Bouchard)
- congenital berry aneurysm
- arteriovenous malformations
- bleeding diseases

      thrombocytopenia

      anticoagulant treatment

      leukaemia

- inflammatory arteritis from whatever cause
- mycotic aneurysm rupture (infective endocarditis)

cerebral embolism

causes

   cardiac

- left atrium

      thrombus in atrial fibrillation

      myxoma

- left ventricle

      myocardial infarction with mural thrombus

      cardiomyopathy

- mitral valve

    rheumatic disease

    infective endocarditis

    prolapse

    prosthesis

- aortic valve

    rheumatic disease

    infective endocarditis

    prosthesis

    atheroma

    syphilis

- *non-cardiac*

    carotid artery atheroma in the neck

    atheroma internal carotid artery siphon in the skull

    atheroma vertebrobasilar arteries

risk factors

- age
- high blood pressure
- cigarette smoking
- positive family history
- hypercholesterolaemia
- peripheral vascular disease
- diabetes
- polycythaemic conditions
- ischaemic heart disease
- atrial fibrillation
- oral contraceptives
- previous transient ischaemic attacks are also an important risk factor

role of high blood pressure

- important risk factor for both haemorrhage and infarction

- risk applies to both systolic and diastolic pressure
- threefold increase in death from stroke in hypertensives
- although high blood pressure is *a* risk factor, the relationship between it and strokes is not absolutely clear cut
- Black *et al.* (1984)[12] found in a consecutive series of stroke patients admitted to hospital that

    46% had *normal* BP

    26% had high BP untreated

    28% with high BP for which they were being treated

  thus one half of stroke cases had normal BP and in another 28% presumably some control of BP+ had been achieved

  in the same series

    haemorrhagic stroke was more common among untreated hypertensives

    infarction was commoner in treated hypertension

    infarction and haemorrhage were equally prevalent in normotensives

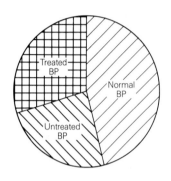

WHO GETS THEM AND WHEN?

age–sex incidence

- as a group strokes are diseases of ageing
- equal incidence in males and females
- however, there are differences in age-incidence

    cerebral infarction – marked increase with age

    cerebral haemorrhage – not infrequent in young and middle-aged

    cerebral embolism – only modest rise with age

    75% of all strokes occur in those aged 65 and over

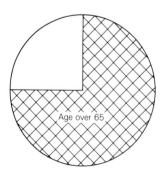

Age	% Strokes
85+	14
75–84	33
65–74	28
	75
55–64	16
45–54	7
below 45	2
	25

frequency

- annual incidence 2–3 per 1000
- point prevalence 5–6 per 1000

general practice

annual cases of strokes in population of 2500

New strokes	5
(death in acute stroke	2)
(resulting severe/moderate disability	2)
Old strokes alive	
in practice	13
(with severe/moderate disability	7)

district general hospital

- approximately 125 000 persons are treated for strokes in NHS hospitals
- 70 000 deaths in UK from strokes (in 1983)
- a DGH will admit about 400 strokes per year and of these up to 200 will die

DGH serving 250 000:

Annual admissions	400
(Deaths	200)
(Severely disabled	100)
(Minor/not disabled	100)
Old strokes in DGH area	1250
(Severely disabled	650)

WHAT HAPPENS?

mortality

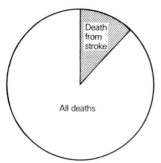

- approximately 70 000 deaths from strokes in UK per year (12% of all deaths)

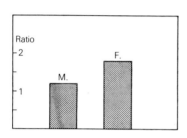

- although the *incidence* of strokes is roughly equal in males and females, the *mortality* is higher in females (M : F = 1.2 : 1.8)

mortality trends

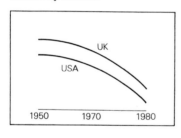

- in developed countries the mortality rates from strokes have been falling

    from 1950 to 1970 slowly

    from 1970 to 1980 quickly

- rates of fall have been faster in USA than in UK
- falls began before introduction of effective antihypertensive drugs

outcomes

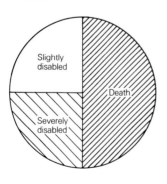

- between 40% and 50% of acute strokes *die* within the first month
- of the *survivors*

    one half severely disabled – mostly hemiplegias

    one half slight or no disabilities

    up to one half of TIAs develop major strokes in 5 years if untreated

WHAT TO DO?

issues

- most strokes (75%) are in over-65s and are part of ageing process
- death rates from strokes are falling all over the world – exact reasons are uncertain
- biggest impact comes from *prevention*
    control of high BP especially in those under 60

    stop smoking

    avoidance of other 'risk factors'
- *acute stroke*
    keep alive

    treat any treatable conditions
- *after stroke*
    rehabilitation, to restore optimal function

diagnosis

- clinical presentation
    transient ischaemic attacks

    cerebral infarction

    cerebral haemorrhage

    multi-infarct dementia

transient ischaemic attacks (TIA)

- important because they lead to full strokes in up to half in 5 years if untreated
- defined as causing symptoms for less than 24 hours
- most originate in atheromatous carotid arteries in the neck (especially at bifurcation common carotid)
- 30% have potential cardiac source of embolism
- may last seconds, minutes, hours – most not longer than 1 hour

- *symptoms*

    carotid territory (Figure 3.1)

    vertebrobasilar territory (Figure 3.2)

- *signs*

    there are often no neurological signs since the patient is usually examined after the attack is over

    there may be signs of the predisposing factors (Figure 3.3)

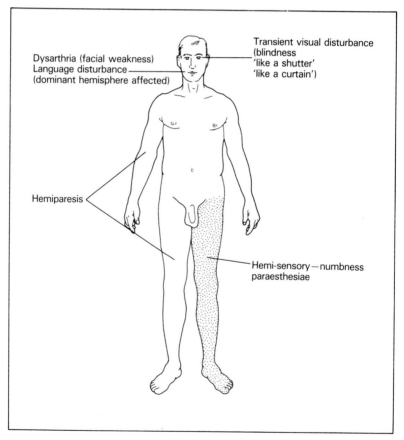

Dysarthria (facial weakness)
Language disturbance
(dominant hemisphere affected)

Transient visual disturbance
(blindness
'like a shutter'
'like a curtain')

Hemiparesis

Hemi-sensory—numbness
paraesthesiae

Figure 3.1   *Symptoms of transient ischaemic attacks in carotid territory*

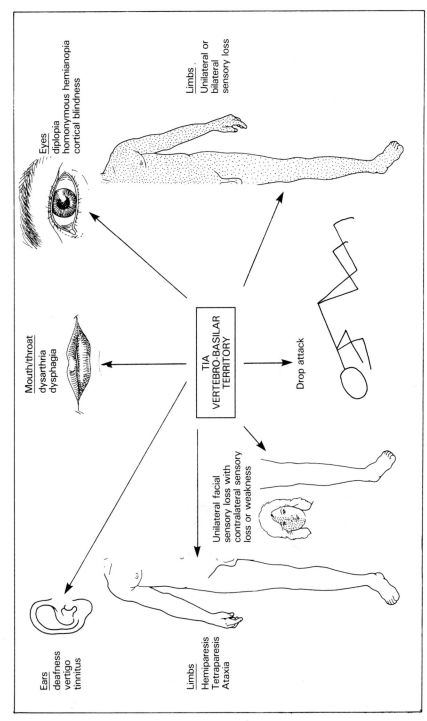

Figure 3.2 *Symptoms in transient ischaemic attacks in vertebrobasilar territory*

Eyes
diplopia
homonymous hemianopia
cortical blindness

Limbs
Unilateral or
bilateral
sensory loss

Mouth/throat
dysarthria
dysphagia

TIA
VERTEBRO-BASILAR
TERRITORY

Drop attack

Unilateral facial
sensory loss with
contralateral sensory
loss or weakness

Ears
deafness
vertigo
tinnitus

Limbs
Hemiparesis
Tetraparesis
Ataxia

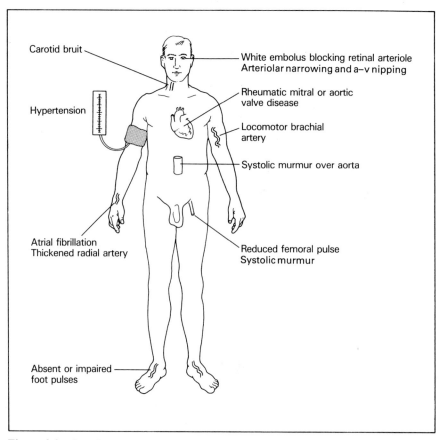

Carotid bruit

White embolus blocking retinal arteriole
Arteriolar narrowing and a–v nipping

Hypertension

Rheumatic mitral or aortic
valve disease

Locomotor brachial
artery

Systolic murmur over aorta

Atrial fibrillation
Thickened radial artery

Reduced femoral pulse
Systolic murmur

Absent or impaired
foot pulses

Figure 3.3   *Possible findings in transient ischaemic attack*

investigations

- aims

    establish cause

    prevent recurrence

    exclude other causes of transient
    neurological disturbances

- blood tests

    Hb and PCV – polycythaemia → thrombosis

    platelets – thrombocythaemia → thrombosis

    ESR ↑ – arteritis → thrombosis

sugar ↑ – diabetes → predisposes to atheroma

lipids ↑ – hyperlipidaemia → predisposes to atheroma

- chest X-ray – rheumatic heart disease
- e.c.g.

    atrial fibrillation → emboli

    myocardial infarction (silent) → emboli

- echocardiogram

    rheumatic heart disease → emboli

    infective endocarditis → emboli

    prolapsed mitral valve → emboli

- arteriography – definitive test: more useful in carotid than vertebrobasilar territory

    indications

    medical control failed

    ischaemic attacks incapacitating

    no significant hypertension

    there is a possibility of surgery

    the patient is fit for surgery

    experienced radiologist

    experienced anaesthetist

    experienced surgeon

- phonoangiography and pulsed Doppler ultrasonic imaging – advanced techniques – special neurological units only
- CT scan – the main value is excluding other causes of transient neurological deficits
- nuclear magnetic resonance (NMR) – a more sophisticated imaging technique which may be superior to CT scanning in showing structural lesions in organs and also functional (chemical) disturbances.

N.B. Not all these investigations are necessary in all cases but it is important not to neglect TIAs

cerebral infarction

- may be preceded by transient ischaemic attacks (up to one in two may develop a stroke within 5 years)
- often premonitory headache for few days
- patient may awaken with a stroke
- loss of consciousness rare
- the typical presentation (middle cerebral artery) is shown in Figure 3.4

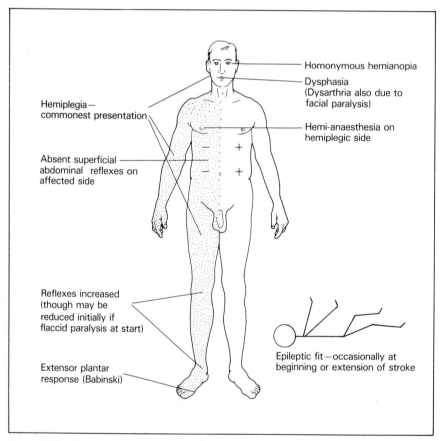

Figure 3.4 *Commonest presentation of cerebral infarction (middle cerebral artery)*

- other presentations may occur

    anterior cerebral

        hemiplegia – leg > arm

        apraxia

        motor dysphasia

        disorder of micturition

    posterior cerebral

        homonymous hemianopia (macula spared)

        burning pain on one side of body (thalamic involvement)

        crossed paralysis characteristic – cranial nerve paresis one side, hemiparesis opposite side

        also   double vision

                nystagmus

                vomiting

                vertigo

                ataxia

- progression

    may be maximal at start

    may evolve in 1–2 hours

    may progress for 1–2 days

    may take 1–2 weeks – suggests internal carotid artery occlusion

    may be stepwise – periodic deterioration with static intervals between.

investigation

- *aims*

    confirm a doubtful clinical diagnosis

    discover any treatable cause

    detect any reversible risk factors

    provide baseline for future assessment

- *CT scan*

    most useful test to establish diagnosis

    shows infarcts > 0.5 cm diameter

    may take 1–2 days to show and may
    disappear after 3–4 weeks

- *e.e.g.*

    of little value because abnormalities are
    non-specific

    may help in assessment of progress – should
    improve, otherwise suspect another cause
    e.g. tumour

- *c.s.f.*

    unnecessary for diagnosis

    potentially hazardous if raised intracranial
    pressure present → coning and death

- *angiography*

    should only be considered if it will influence
    management

    may show an operable carotid artery lesion
    in the neck

    see TIAs (p. 59) for requirements for
    angiography to be considered

cerebral haemorrhage

- strongly associated with hypertension
- majority occur in internal capsule (Figure 3.5)
- onset often abrupt
- usually when awake – unlike cerebral
  infarction
- loss of consciousness in majority
- initial epileptic fit common
- usually produces hemiplegia

    flaccid initially

    spastic later

- raised intracranial pressure often with
  papilloedema
- prognosis poor – 50% die within few days

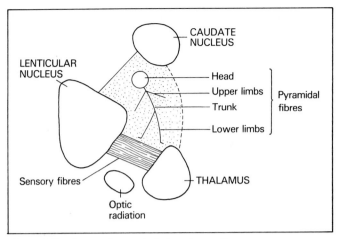

Figure 3.5   *Internal capsule in basal ganglia*

- other possible sites of haemorrhage
    - brain stem
        - hyperpyrexia
        - pinpoint pupils
        - Cheyne–Stokes respiration
        - bilateral involvement of cranial nerves and pyramidal tracts
    - cerebellar
        - occipital headache
        - vomiting
        - vertigo
        - ataxia
        - pupillary constriction
        - contralateral hemiplegia

investigations

- need to investigate is limited
    - probably older patient
    - chances are against recovery anyway
    - results of any tests are unlikely to modify management

- CT scan – best test – can diagnose intracerebral haemorrhage within minutes of onset
- c.s.f. – not very useful – intracerebral haemorrhage can occur without any leak of blood into sub-arachnoid space

multi-infarct dementia

- repeated small cerebral infarcts – 'stepwise' progression
- impairment of memory and intellect
- may evolve into dementia
- findings

    hypertension often

    focal neurological signs

    vascular murmurs especially carotids in neck
- pseudobulbar palsy may be associated

    dysarthria

    dysphasia

    bilateral pyramidal signs

    small stepping gait (*marche à petits pas*)
- diagnosis – CT scan best

management

principles

- treat causal lesion if possible
- protect ischaemic brain from necrosis
- immediate treatment to prevent hazards of unconsciousness in haemorrhagic stroke
- prevention and treatment of complications
- rehabilitation for disabled patients
- prevention of recurrence

causal lesion

- hypertension

    both systolic and diastolic pressures should be reduced

bring pressure down slowly

don't reduce diastolic pressure < 100 mm →
danger of extending infarction

i.m. methyldopa is good agent for
unconscious patient

- cardiac source of embolism

    ensure absence of haemorrhage by CT scan
    if possible

    anticoagulate

- arteritis – treat with steroids

protection of ischaemic brain from necrosis

- reduction of cerebral oedema has been tried
  but convincing evidence of benefit is lacking

- methods to reduce oedema

    dexamethasone orally

    i.v. mannitol

    i.v. glycerol

- other methods have been tried to improve
  cerebral blood supply but are inconclusive

    dextran infusion

    cerebral vasodilators

    inhalation of carbon dioxide

    hyperbaric oxygen

    stellate ganglion block

complications of acute stroke

- bronchopneumonia

    physiotherapy

    care of airways

    antibiotics

    tracheostomy occasionally needed

    mobility as soon as possible

- deep vein thrombosis

    physiotherapy

    mobilize early if possible

    anticoagulants if cerebral haemorrhage excluded

- pulmonary embolus

    frequent cause of death

    treat as for deep vein thrombosis

- pressure sores

    good nursing

    ripple mattress

    early mobilization

- urinary infection

    appliance in males

    catheter in females

    urinary antibiotics

- stiffness and contractures in hemiplegic limits

    active physiotherapy

- depression

    common

    optimistic encouragement – improvement can continue up to 3 years after onset

    antidepressives if necessary

- nutrition

    maintain nutrition

    nasogastric feeding if can't swallow

    i.v. alimentation in unconscious patients

    use vitamin supplements parentally

rehabilitation

- essential to start as early as possible
- means   physiotherapy

            occupational therapy

            speech therapy

- additional help   stroke club

                               day centre care

                               district nurse/health visitor

                               volunteer organization
- retraining courses for suitable patients to return to work

home or hospital?

- 50% of patients in UK treated at home
- indications for hospital

    diagnosis in doubt

    domiciliary aid not available

    unsatisfactory social circumstance

    stroke-unit available in hospital
- acute phase admission may be desirable

    reassure relatives

    rehabilitation started

    domiciliary community services arranged

treatment of transient ischaemic attacks

medical

- aspirin
- dipyridamole (Persantin)
- anticoagulation (Warfarin)
- aspirin

    should be tried first
    prevents platelets clumping by inhibition of thromboxane A_2 produced by platelets

    low dose should be used – 75 mg/day

    active peptic ulcer is contraindication
- dipyramidole

    inhibits platelet clumping by boosting intracellular AMP

    can be used in conjunction with aspirin

    dose 100 mg t.d.s.

- Warfarin

    used when aspirin and dipyridamole fail to control TIAs

    contraindications   severe hypertension

    active peptic ulcer

    bleeding disorder

    liver disease

    side-effect – bleeding in   skin

    muscle

    kidney

    brain

    retroperitoneal (simulates an 'acute abdomen')

surgical   carotid endarterectomy – indications

- failed medical treatment
- incapacitating TIAs
- substantial carotid obstruction ($> 60\%$)
- experienced surgeon available
- contraindications

    myocardial infarction < 6 months

    unstable angina

    severe lung disease

    advanced age

PROGNOSIS OF STROKES

cerebral infarction

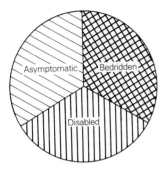

- hospital mortality
    - 30% in 1 month
    - 50% in 6 months
- stroke survivors:
    - one third remain bedridden
    - one third asymptomatic
    - life expectancy halved
    - second stroke   10% within 1 year
    -                      20% within 5 years
    - 3-year mortality 50% from   recurrent stroke
    -   heart attacks

cerebral haemorrhage

- 80% mortality in first month
- adverse prognostic features:
    - impairment of consciousness
    - defects in conjugate gaze
    - severe and persistent hemiplegia
    - Cheyne–Stokes respiration

transient ischaemic attacks

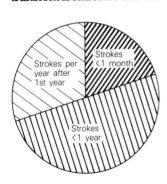

- one in two may develop stroke < 5 years
- 20% strokes within first month
- 50% strokes within first year
- annual incidence after – 5% per year
- after surgery
    - 30% mortality < 5 years
    - 25% recurrence < 5 years

Useful practical points

- don't forget cardiac dysrhythmia, especially atrial fibrillation, as a cause of TIA

- a carotid bruit in the neck suggests the most likely source of emboli in TIAs, but up to 50% of all potentially operable carotid lesions do not have a bruit

- always try medical treatment (aspirin, dipyridamole, warfarin) for TIAs before considering the possibility of surgery

- a lumbar puncture is of very little help in differentiating cerebral infarction from cerebral haemorrhage and may be potentially lethal if there is raised intracranial pressure

- A CT scan is the best test available for diagnosing a cerebral infarct or haemorrhage and supersedes all other tests

- prevention by control of high blood pressure is most hopeful, but this will prevent less than one half of all strokes

4   ASTHMA

WHAT IS IT?

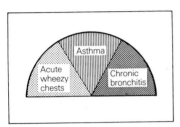

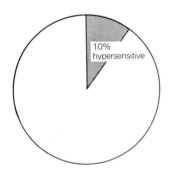

- a definition of *asthma* is difficult: essentially it is a transient obstruction of the small airways due to a variety of causes: the clinical manifestation is recurrent episodes of wheezing and breathlessness

- the *spectrum* ranges widely and within it there are three useful clinical groupings

    'acute wheezy chests' in children (AWC)

    'true asthma' at all ages

    acute wheezy episodes in 'chronic bronchitis' associated with varying degrees of permanent obstruction (chronic obstructive airways disease – COAD)

- it is likely that there is a predisposing *diathesis* in about 10% of the population who have hypersensitive or hyperreactive bronchioles associated with asthma

WHO GETS IT AND WHEN?

age

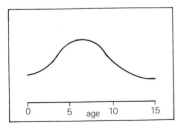

accepting the widest definition of 'asthma' there are different patterns of *age-prevalence* in the three types

- *acute wheezy chests in children* – maximal in early childhood, peak at 4–8 years and then decline

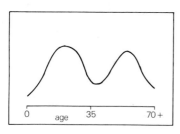

- asthma (adult onset) – there are two peaks of prevalence in early adult life and in late life

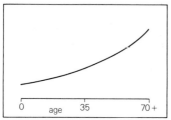

- chronic bronchitic 'wheezers' rise with age

sex

- prevalence rates
    - in young M>F
    - in middle age F>M
    - in elderly M=F

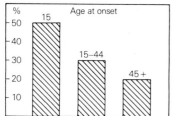

- in one half of asthmatics, attacks start in childhood
    - in one third at 15–44
    - in one fifth after 45

frequency

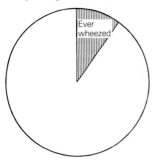

- 100 per 1000 (10%) of population *have had* bouts of chest wheezing

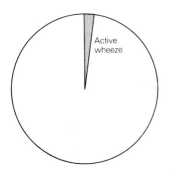
Active
wheeze

- between ten and 20 per 1000 *have* wheezy attacks (asthma) in any year

general practice

asthma in general practice population 2500:

Annual new cases (incidence)	2–3
Annual attacks	35 persons (50 attacks)
Past and present asthmatics (wheezers)	250
Death from asthma	1 in 15 years (1 per 750 attacks of asthma)

district general hospital

asthma in DGH with population of 250 000:

Annual admissions	250
Attending OPDs	1000
Deaths from asthma in district per year	7*

* how many of these seven deaths are preventable?

atopic (intrinsic) and non-atopic (extrinsic) asthma

the distinctive features are:

- atopic

    early onset

    episodic attacks

    family history of allergic disorder

- non-atopic

  late onset

  chronic symptoms

  severe attacks more likely

  no family history

associated features

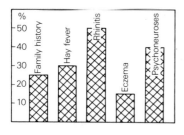

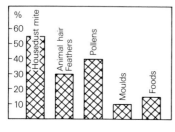

- family history +ve in 25% – mainly in atopic asthma

- hay fever – 30% (7% in non-asthmatic population)

- 'rhinitis' – 20%

- eczema – 15% (5% in non-asthmatic population)

- psychoneuroses – 40% (12% in non-asthmatic population)

- *allergens* (more than one per asthmatic are possible)

  housedust mite – 55%

  animal hair, feathers – 30%

  pollens – 40%

  moulds – 10%

  foods – 15%

WHAT HAPPENS?

- the *general outlook* for uncomplicated asthma is good – in majority attacks cease or are mild and infrequent

- a pattern appears to be that there is a *'period of activity'* with attacks for 10–20 years followed by natural remission

ASTHMA

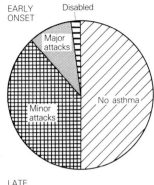

EARLY ONSET

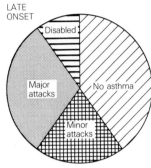

LATE ONSET

- *factors*

  early onset – better prognosis (<15 years)

	Onset: age	
	<15 years	>15 years
No attacks of asthma	50	40
Minor	38	20
Major	10	30
Disabled +	2	10
	100	100

(Data: ref. 1)

- *allergies in wheezy children: at 15 years*
  - *children with no allergies* – no asthma in 63%
  - children *with allergies* – no asthma in 20%

history

symptoms

- episodic attacks of chest tightness, wheezing and breathlessness
- diurnal variation is an important diagnostic feature – always worse in early hours and on waking
- chronic breathlessness with wheezing most days and nights
- sometimes recurrent cough worse at night may be the only symptom
- growth failure may occur in children with chronic asthma
- susceptibility to respiratory infections

trigger factors

- bronchial hypersensitivity

    cold air

    smoke/fumes

    aerosols

- drugs

    salicylates

    non-steroidal anti-inflammatory drugs

    tartrazine dyes in food

- emotional disturbances

- exercise – especially in children

physical signs   physical signs are shown in Figure 4.1

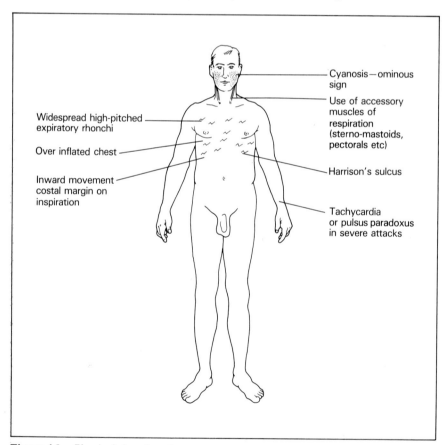

Figure 4.1   *Physical signs in asthma*

differential diagnosis

- the main differential diagnosis is between asthma and chronic bronchitis – the distinctive features in asthma are:

    childhood symptoms often

    family history especially in atopic asthma

    non-smoker usually

    nocturnal attacks

    morning tightness in the chest

- differentiation from left ventricular failure (cardiac asthma)

	Asthma	Left vent. failure
Past history	asthma respiratory infections	high blood pressure angina or heart attack valvular disease
Timing	early morning	any time
Breathlessness	expiratory	inspiratory
Cough	before dyspnoea	after dyspnoea
Sputum	thick, gelatinous	pink, frothy
Relief	bronchodilator	diuretic
Signs	mainly rhonchi	mainly crepitations

- large airway obstruction (e.g. bronchial cancer) – the two main distinguishing points are:

    absence of morning tightness

    difficulty with inspiration rather than expiration

WHAT TO DO?

issues

- asthma is a very distressing disease in childhood and may have profound effects in disrupting education and social life

- although in some cases the cause may be known and the precipitating factor identifiable, in many cases attacks occur 'out of the blue' so no effective prophylactic treatment is possible

- attacks of asthma can be aborted by effective and *early* treatment and in those patients responding the prognosis is good

- in some patients, however, failure to respond to the standard treatment can lead to a critical condition and life may be endangered

- it is incumbent upon the doctor to identify and arrange urgent hospital treatment for patients with life-threatening asthma; but it is just as important for the patient to be educated enough about his condition to seek medical aid at these times

- the prognosis in 75% of children with asthma is good, so an optimistic outlook can be offered to the child and his parents

investigations

respiratory function tests

- these are the most helpful tests in asthma

- the measurements required are

    one-second forced expiratory volume (FEV_1) – spirometer (Figure 4.2)

    peak expiratory flow – this is the easiest test and the patient should be taught to do this on a mini-peak flow meter at home – several measurements during the day are much more helpful than a single one

- reversibility of small airway obstruction with a bronchodilator aerosol is a useful diagnostic test in asthma, but may be variable according to the severity of the asthma

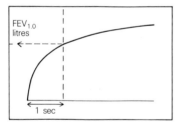

Figure 4.2 *Spirometer trace showing FEV_1*

- regular measurements of peak flow are helpful both in diagnosis of asthma and in assessing the response to treatment
- an early morning dip in the peak expiratory flow is an important diagnostic sign of asthma
- a similar fall in peak expiratory flow can often be shown after vigorous exercise in asthmatics, especially in children, and is also diagnostic of asthma

skin tests of allergy

these are seldom helpful and rarely relevant in the management of asthma. They should not be done as a routine

chest X-ray

this is usually normal in asthma and should not be done routinely. It is indicated if a pneumothorax is suspected in an acute attack

blood tests

although eosinophilia may be present with a raised IgE in asthma this is rarely of diagnostic value and so it is not necessary to do these tests as a routine

provocation tests

the response to intranasal or intrabronchial challenge with histamine, methacholine or other allergens is potentially dangerous and rarely necessary, except perhaps in cases of suspected occupational asthma

deaths from asthma

- sudden and unexpected after a short attack
- chronic asthmatics with a long and troublesome past history
- fatal attack resulting from an underestimate of severity and therefore inadequacy of treatment
- underuse of steroids – used either too late or in an inadequate dose
- recently discharged from hospital

treatment

general measures
- educate patient/relatives
  - nature of asthma
  - likely causes
  - when to seek medical help
- counselling for emotional problems
- train to use peak flow meter
- avoidance of allergens where possible
- desensitization – rarely effective
- exercise programme, especially swimming – bronchodilator or cromoglycate prior to exercise may help performance
- treat respiratory infections promptly with antibiotics

specific treatment

The drugs available are
- bronchodilator aerosols
- methylxanthines
- cromoglycate
- steroids

bronchodilator aerosols

β_2 stimulants

    salbutamol (Ventolin) 2 puffs (200 μg) 4–6-hourly

    terbutaline (Bricanyl) 1 – 2 puffs (250–500 μg) 4–6-hourly

    rimiterol (Pulmadil) 1–3 puffs (200–600 μg) up to 3-hourly

    tenoterol (Berotec) 1–2 puffs (200–400 μg) 4–6-hourly

sympathomimetic

    isoprenaline (Medihaler) 1–3 puffs (80–240 μg) – up to 3-hourly

    orciprenaline (Alupent) 1–2 puffs (670–1340 μg) – up to 2-hourly

anticholinergic

    ipratropium (Atrovent) 1–2 puffs (18–36 μg) 4-hourly

---

methylxanthines

---

aminophylline

    i.v. 5 mg/kg bolus

    0.9 mg/kg per hour infusion

    tablets: 100–300 mg repeated p.r.n.

choline theophyllinate (Choledyl)

    200 mg t.d.s. (8 mg/kg)

    6-hourly in children

theophylline (Nuelin)

    60–250 mg 3–4 times daily

    5 – 6 mg/kg 6-hourly in children

---

methylxanthines are generally less effective
bronchodilators than the aerosols – the
indications for their use are:

    very mild asthma

    patients unable to use an aerosol

    nocturnal symptoms in spite of cromoglycate
    and steroid aerosols

sodium cromoglycate (Intal)
This drug helps to stabilize the mast cells in the
lungs and so prevent an allergic antigen–antibody
reaction leading to bronchospasm. It is therefore
solely of prophylactic value and cannot be used to
control an acute attack. It is most useful in:

    childhood asthma

    extrinsic (atopic) asthma

    exercise induced asthma

steroids
These can be used as aerosols or tablets

	Aerosol	Tablet
Advantages	smaller dose	larger dose possible for more severe cases
	direct bronchial contact no systemic absorption	easier than aerosol for some patients
Disadvantages	husky voice candidiasis	side-effects: fluid retention oedema weight gain increased BP potassium loss hyperglycaemia

preparations available

aerosol

    beclomethasone (Becotide) 2 puffs (100 μg) q.d.s.

    betamethasone (Bextasol) 2 puffs (200 μg) q.d.s.

oral prednisolone

  acute attack

    30–60 mg/day to start

    reduce by 5 mg/day

    long term – 2.5–7.5 mg/day

treatment of an acute attack of asthma

- mild

    bronchodilator

        > 8 years age – aerosol

        < 8 years age – oral e.g. salbutamol 1–2 mg t.d.s.

    theophylline tablets

- moderate

    bronchodilator

      metered aerosol

      hand nebulizer (air cylinder or compression pump)

theophylline tablets

aminophylline suppository

s.c. terbutaline   250–500 μg 2–4/day

child 10 μg/kg

- severe – hospital admission is usually desirable

note – each district should have urgent admission policy for severe asthma which if necessary can bypass GP

diagnosis of a severe attack

- can't lie down because of breathlessness
- bed/chair held to fix shoulder girdle
- unable to talk
- pale and sweating
- tachycardia
- pulsus paradoxus

signs of impending disaster   these signs are shown in Figure 4.3

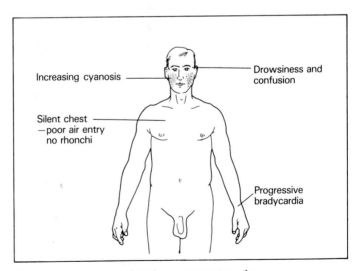

Increasing cyanosis

Drowsiness and confusion

Silent chest
—poor air entry
no rhonchi

Progressive bradycardia

Figure 4.3   *Ominous signs in severe acute asthma*

hospital management

tests required

- chest X-ray to exclude pneumothorax
- arterial sample for P_{O_2}, P_{CO_2}, pH
- venous sample for serum potassium
- lung function tests no use

treatment

- intravenous aminophylline bolus 5 mg/kg
  infuse 0.9 mg/kg per hour
- intravenous hydrocortisone 2.5 mg/kg
  every 2 hours
- bronchodilator inhalation 2–4-hourly by
  nebulizer driven by oxygen or compression
  pump
- continuous oxygen
- intravenous fluid and potassium
  replacement
- oral prednisolone

  100 mg in first 12 h

  20–40 mg/day for 7–10 days

  DO NOT SEDATE

  assessment of response

- clinical improvement
- heart rate return to normal
- P_{O_2} rises to normal

  indications for assisted ventilation

- continued clinical deterioration

  acute respiratory distress

  extreme exhaustion

  hypotension

  increasing bradycardia

  increasing cyanosis

- $P_a{O_2}$ falls below 6.5 kPa
- P_{CO_2} rises above 6.5 kPa

long term management of asthma

- if attacks infrequent, no interval treatment required
- if attacks frequent

    bronchodilator

    > 8 years old – aerosol

    < 8 years old – tablets

    oral theophylline

    cromoglycate regularly q.d.s.

- indications for steroids

    inadequate response to triple therapy above

    recurrent nocturnal asthma

    prolongation of morning tightness through the day

    quality of life impaired

- it may be desirable to provide bad asthmatics with a supply of oral prednisolone to use on their own initiative for a severe exacerbation not responding to bronchodilators, ensuring that they are fully conversant with its use beforehand

- administration of steroids

    continue triple therapy

    metered aerosol > 8 years of age

    dry powder (Becotide Rotacap) 4–8 years of age

    oral prednisolone – use if steroid aerosol ineffective in a dose of 16 puffs/day – start with 5–10 mg/day and reduce if possible by 1 mg every month to smallest effective daily maintenance dose

    watch out for side-effects

    fluid retention   weight gain

    oedema

    hypertension

        potassium loss   weakness

                             cardiac arrhythmias

     hyperglycaemia

- ACTH/Synacthen – sole indication is for children with stunted growth not responding to cromoglycate and inhaled steroids

---

Pitfalls

- mislabelling an asthmatic child as 'bronchitis' and treating with antibiotics only, so depriving it of the benefits of bronchodilator treatment

- the use of steroid aerosols for trivial asthma

- the use of cromoglycate to control an acute attack

- failure to use a sympathomimetic bronchodilator aerosol before starting treatment with a steroid aerosol

- failure to check thoroughly whether the patient has the correct technique for aerosol inhalation

- the use of combination products such as cromoglycate/beclomethasone as initial therapy

---

Useful practical points

- in bronchial asthma the respiratory difficulty is primarily expiratory and in cardiac asthma it is inspiratory: the response to a bronchodilator aerosol will also help to distinguish the two

- less than 25% of children with asthma will still continue with severe symptoms in adult life

- although there is generally a good prognosis in that over 50% of patients either stop having attacks or are minimally inconvenienced, patients still die of asthma and it is important to recognize the danger signs and refer the patient for urgent hospital treatment. –

  drowsiness and confusion

  increasing cyanosis

  silent chest

  progressive bradycardia

- in severe asthma it is best to assess progress objectively by simple respiratory tests such as peak expiratory flow: the most useful test in hospital is analysis of blood gases (PCO_2, PO_2)

- with the current available drugs most active asthmatics can be relieved and attacks controlled; nevertheless there is need for each district to have policies for management of the dangerous severe acute attack

5   CHRONIC BRONCHITIS

WHAT IS IT?

- defined as 'daily cough with sputum for at least 3 months for 2 consecutive years'
- it is more than this – a syndrome that may include

    cough and sputum

    bouts of acute chest infection with wheezing and other abnormal chest signs

    breathlessness

    various degrees of respiratory insufficiency
- causes are multiple and indefinite

    cigarette smoking – most important

    atmospheric pollution and climate

    certain occupations

    recurring infections

    genetic (familial) predisposition

    asthma and other chest disorders

pathological features

- hypersecretion of mucus from hypertrophic bronchial glands
- inflammatory changes from infection
- narrowing of bronchial/bronchiolar airways
- emphysema
- pulmonary hypertension
- cardiac failure

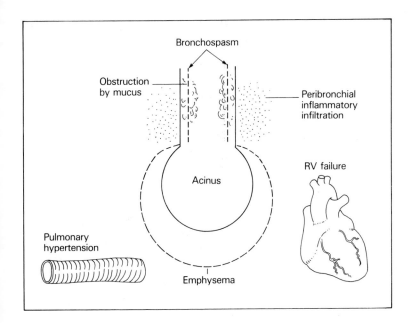

three clinical types

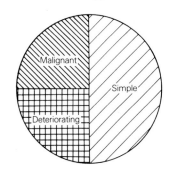

- *simple* with cough/sputum but little or no functional disability (50%)

- *deteriorating* with moderate disability and recurring infection (25%)

- *malignant* – progressive severe disability with respiratory failure (25%)

WHO, WHEN AND WHERE?

- *'chronic bronchitis'* has been known as the 'British disease' because the highest mortality rates are in UK – but this may be due more to customs of diagnostic 'disease-labelling' than to real differences. (In other countries it may be labelled as 'asthma' or 'sinusitis')

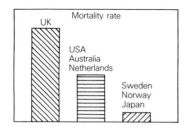
Mortality rate

UK

USA
Australia
Netherlands

Sweden
Norway
Japan

- *mortality rates* in UK are twice as high as in USA etc, and ten times higher than in Sweden etc[15]

- in UK highest mortality rates in Northern Ireland, Scotland, North of England and Wales and lowest in South

- *age – sex*

    prevalence increases with age

    M>F

- *social class*

    more prevalent in lower social classes

- very much a *general practice disease* – where all but the most severe cases are managed

- *prevalence*

    10% of UK population, i.e. 5–6 million, have chronic bronchitis

    20–30% of adults (over 40) have chronic bronchitis

    in any year 4% of population (2.5 million) will receive medical treatment for chronic bronchitis in UK

- *annual deaths in UK* (certified as chronic bronchitis)

    30 000 (true figure probably double, since death certificates often state other causes such as 'heart failure' or 'pneumonia')

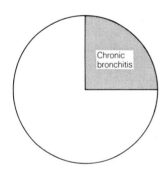
Chronic bronchitis

general practice	chronic bronchitis in a practice population of 2500 per year	
	Cases of chronic bronchitis (prevalence)	250
	Annual patients consulting (simple: 60) (acute infection: 30) (respiratory invalids: 10)	100
	Admitted to hospital	5
	Deaths	1–2
district general hospital	DGH serving 250 000 population	
	Total cases of chronic bronchitis per 250 000	25 000
	Annual acute and other admissions	500
	Attending outpatient departments	1500 (?)

- hospitals see only the tip of the chronic bronchitis iceberg and see only the more severe cases

WHAT HAPPENS?

natural history

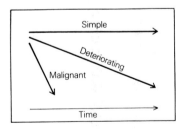

- one half of chronic bronchitics are '*simple*', life expectancy *not* shortened and without very much disability apart from productive cough

- one quarter slow and progressive *deterioration* of respiratory function with breathlessness and acute attacks of infection

- one quarter become severely disabled – *respiratory invalids* .

prognosis

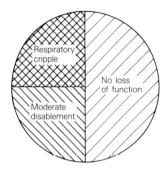

- one half will be minimally affected with very little functional disability
- one quarter will be moderately disabled with restriction of work and leisure activities
- one quarter will deteriorate rapidly and die within 5–10 years of onset of symptoms
- factors influencing prognosis

    'pink puffers' are less prone to respiratory infection than are 'blue bloaters'

    respiratory failure more likely in a 'pink puffer'

    onset of cor pulmonale has very adverse effect on prognosis – patients die within 2–3 years

    degree of impairment of FEV_1 is good guide to prognosis

clinical presentation

the three cardinal symptoms are

- cough
- sputum
- breathlessness

simple chronic bronchitis

history

- cough

    at first only in morning

    often after first cigarette

    gradually more persistent

- sputum

    usually mucoid

    easily purulent with infection

    continuous through the day

    haemoptysis very rare – always consider

    TB

    cancer

    bronchiectasis

CHRONIC BRONCHITIS

- breathlessness

    initially only on effort

    variable

    worse on cold or foggy day

    gradually worsens until

      on dressing/undressing

      walking about house

      getting in/out bed

    may occur at night with coughing –
    distinguish from pulmonary oedema

	Chronic bronchitis	Pulmonary oedema (cardiac asthma)
Dyspnoea	expiratory	inspiratory
Cough	before dyspnoea	after dyspnoea
Sputum	thick, gelatinous purulent	pink, frothy
Relief	coughing up sputum	standing up
Lung signs	mainly rhonchi	mainly fine crepitations
Heart signs	nil	gallop rhythm

- wheezing

    on exertion

    after coughing bout

    on lying down

- chest pain – only if associated pleurisy

examination – the signs in uncomplicated chronic bronchitis are minimal

- none in mild disease

- scattered rhonchi – inspiratory, expiratory

- wheezing after paroxysm of coughing

- scattered coarse crepitations in severe disease

acute on chronic bronchitis

periodic exacerbations of chronic bronchitis

- often follow viral infections of respiratory tract, especially winter
- cough and breathlessness become worse
- sputum becomes purulent

    green

    yellow

- wheezing often develops

examination

- fever may be present
- increase in rhonchi
- may be localized area of crepitations due to bacterial pneumonia

severe complicated disease

the major complications are

- severe emphysema ('pink puffer')
- cor pulmonale ('blue bloater')
- cardiorespiratory failure

    'pink puffer'

    the predominant pathology is emphysema

    the signs are shown in Figure 5.1

    'blue bloater'

    the predominant pathology is

    RV failure

    chronic bronchitis

    the signs are shown in Figure 5.2

    there is often a mixed picture with features of both

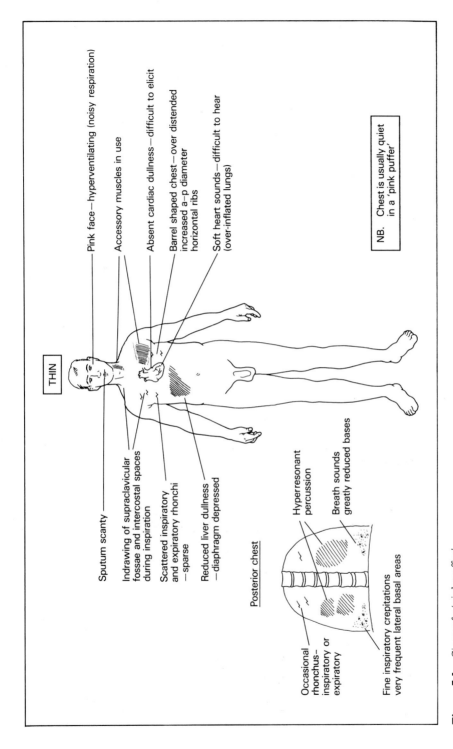

Figure 5.1 *Signs of a 'pink puffer'*

THIN

Pink face—hyperventilating (noisy respiration)

Accessory muscles in use

Absent cardiac dullness—difficult to elicit

Barrel shaped chest—over distended
increased a–p diameter
horizontal ribs

Soft heart sounds—difficult to hear
(over-inflated lungs)

NB. Chest is usually quiet
in a 'pink puffer'

Sputum scanty

Indrawing of supraclavicular
fossae and intercostal spaces
during inspiration

Scattered inspiratory
and expiratory rhonchi
—sparse

Reduced liver dullness
—diaphragm depressed

Posterior chest

Hyperresonant
percussion

Breath sounds
greatly reduced bases

Occasional
rhonchus–
inspiratory or
expiratory

Fine inspiratory crepitations
very frequent lateral basal areas

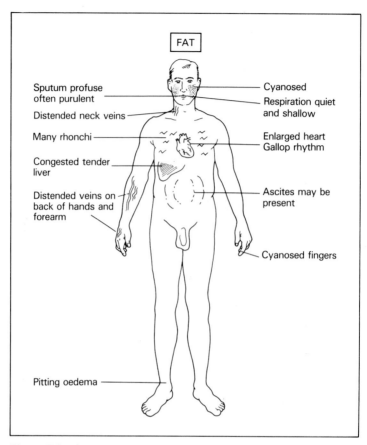

Figure 5.2 *Signs of a 'blue bloater'*

- the clinical differences between the pink puffer and blue bloater are summarized in the table

	Pink puffer	*Blue bloater*
Colour	pink	blue
Breathing	heavy, noisy	quiet, shallow
Sputum	scanty, mucoid	profuse, purulent
R. heart failure	absent	present
Chest infections	few	very susceptible
Respiratory failure	rare but serious	frequent
Prognosis	fair	bad

respiratory failure

- commonest pulmonary cause of ventilatory failure is chronic bronchitis
- defined objectively as

    $PCO_2 > 45$ mm (6.0 kPa)

    $PO_2 < 60$ mm (8 kPa)

- often precipitated by infection
- presentation

    dyspnoea – may be absent if poor ventilatory drive as in the 'blue bloater'

    episodic apnoea during sleep

    drowsiness and confusion, agitation

    headache (CO_2 retention)

    inability to concentrate

    c.v.s.

       warm limbs

       rapid bounding pulse

       cardiac arrhythmia, e.g. atrial fibrillation

       hypotension

       eventually circulatory collapse

    fundi

       congested veins

       papilloedema – less common

    flapping tremor, muscle twitching

- diagnosis – blood gas measurements (see above)
- requires urgent hospital admission and treatment, probably with assisted ventilation

WHAT TO DO?

issues

- very common condition
- multifactorial due to chronic irritation of susceptible respiratory tract from

    smoking

    atmospheric pollution and climate

    occupational hazards

- long course with appreciable disability and mortality
- although there is much that can be done to relieve the effects the main hope is prevention *through avoiding smoking* and improving the atmosphere

differential diagnosis

chronic asthma

- long history of episodic attacks of wheezing starting in childhood
- past history of hay fever or eczema
- family history of asthma or hay fever
- often non-smokers (given up early)
- chest examination

    no attack – no signs

    attack

    accessory muscles used

    high pitched expiratory rhonchi + +

- tests

    blood – eosinophilia

    sputum – eosinophils

    chest X-ray

    may be normal

    may show hyperinflation only

    respiratory function

    reversible small airway obstruction

    no restrictive defect

- therapeutic trials may help in differentiation

    trial of bronchodilator

    trial of steroids – more effective in asthma

tuberculosis

- history of contact with TB
- fever and night sweats
- haemoptysis

- chest examination

    there may be no signs

    see Figure 5.3 for possible signs

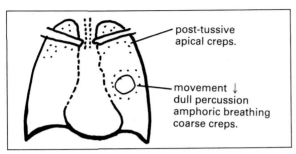

post-tussive
apical creps.

movement ↓
dull percussion
amphoric breathing
coarse creps.

Figure 5.3 *Possible signs in pulmonary tuberculosis with cavitation*

- tests

    chest X-ray

    repeated sputum for tubercle bacilli

bronchiectasis

- past history of severe measles/whooping cough
- lung trouble going back to childhood
- profuse offensive purulent sputum

    on getting up in morning

    on any change in posture

- haemoptysis
- examination (Figure 5.4)

    finger clubbing

    coarse crepitations – often basal

    associated   fibrosis

                            collapse

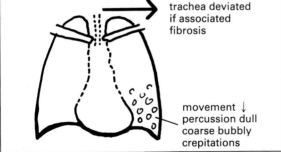

trachea deviated
if associated
fibrosis

movement ↓
percussion dull
coarse bubbly
crepitations

Figure 5.4 *Possible signs in bronchiectasis*

- amyloidosis if longstanding leading to

  oedema

  diarrhoea
- tests

  chest X-ray will distinguish

  bronchogram not justified unless surgery
  contemplated

cancer of bronchus

- only recent cough (unless superimposed on
  chronic bronchitis)
- haemoptysis frequent
- anorexia and loss of weight marked
- metastatic

  brain   headache

             fits

             focal neurological signs

             papilloedema

  bone – pain, fractures

  liver – enlarged, painful

  mediastinal obstruction
- non-metastatic

  peripheral neuropathy

  cerebellar degeneration

  muscle involvement   weakness

                         pain

  Cushing's syndrome
- examination – see Figure 5.5
- tests

  chest X-ray

  bronchoscopy (mandatory)

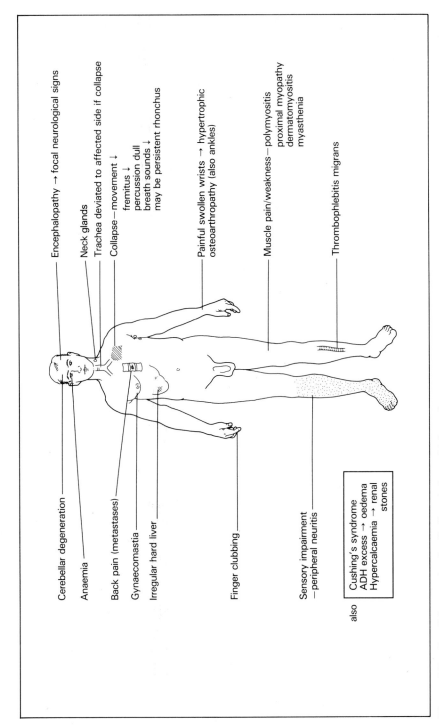

Cerebellar degeneration

Anaemia

Back pain (metastases)

Gynaecomastia

Irregular hard liver

Finger clubbing

Sensory impairment
—peripheral neuritis

also | Cushing's syndrome
ADH excess → oedema
Hypercalcaemia → renal
stones

Encephalopathy → focal neurological signs

Neck glands

Trachea deviated to affected side if collapse

Collapse—movement ↓
fremitus ↓
percussion dull
breath sounds ↓
may be persistent rhonchus

Painful swollen wrists → hypertrophic
osteoarthropathy (also ankles)

Muscle pain/weakness—polymyositis
proximal myopathy
dermatomyositis
myasthenia

Thrombophlebitis migrans

Figure 5.5   *Possible examination findings in bronchial carcinoma*

pneumoconiosis

- many occupations

  miner – silicosis

  aircraft industry – berylliosis

  building – asbestosis

  textiles – byssinosis

  farming – 'farmer's lung'

- long exposure required
- very little respiratory disability for a long time
- sputum often black in miners
- frequently coexists with chronic bronchitis
- chest signs minimal or absent unless advanced fibrosis in late stages
- respiratory function tests – very little impairment
- chest X-ray

  fine nodulation

  nodular opacities

  massive fibrosis

  cavitation may occur but don't forget TB which can develop

- tuberculosis is a not uncommon complication

investigations

chest X-ray

- may be normal
- increased bronchovascular markings at lung bases
- prominent pulmonary artery
- old scars of infections may occur
- large heart if cor pulmonale
- emphysema often – see Figure 5.6

  overtranslucent

  low flat diaphragm

  horizontal ribs

  bullae may be present

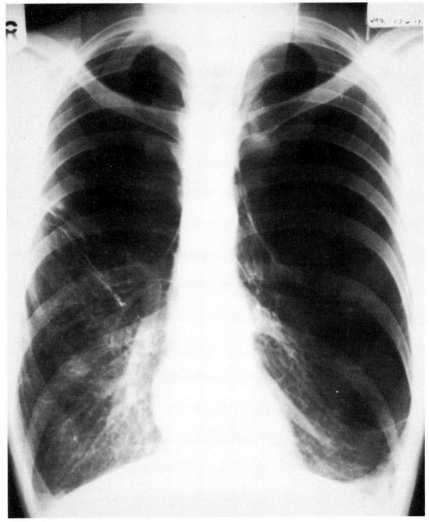

Figure 5.6   *Chest X-ray showing overtranslucent lungs, horizontal ribs and low flat diaphragm in emphysema*

respiratory function tests

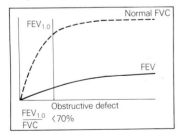

- very useful test with Vitalograph
- peak flow meter (or mini-meter) very useful to assess patient's progress at home
- obstructive defect usually found
- reversibility of small air obstruction can be tested – useful in deciding treatment with bronchodilators

blood gases (Pco_2 and Po_2)	• very useful measurements in assessing severe disease
	• mandatory if suspected respiratory failure
	• useful in following response to treatment
sputum	• can be examined for bacteria
	• very little diagnostic help
	• usually sterile
	• result arrives too late to decide initial treatment
	• may be useful in patients resistant to antibiotics
	• very limited value in picking up malignant cells
	• mandatory if TB suspected
e.c.g.	• helpful test in deciding cor pulmonale – shows right ventricular hypertrophy (Figure 5.7)
	right axis deviation in limb leads
	tall R in VI
	ST depression and T inversion if RV strain has developed
blood count	• secondary polycythaemia
	increased Hb
	increased red cells
	increased packed cell volume
	• leukocytosis – if active bacterial infection

TREATMENT

principles

- general measures
- specific measures
  - infection
  - airway obstruction

anoxaemia

heart failure

- rehabilitation

general measures • the most important is stopping smoking

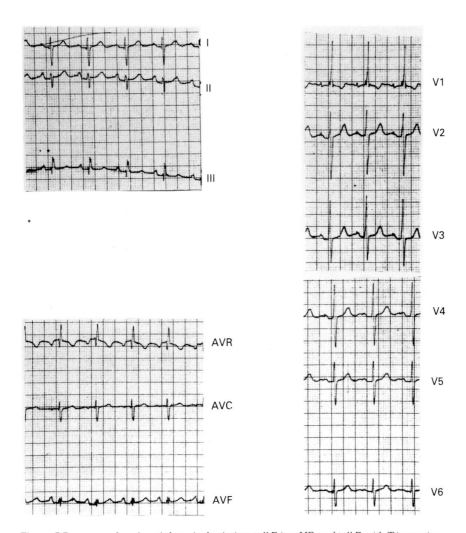

Figure 5.7 *e.c.g. showing right axis deviation, tall R in a VR and tall R with T inversion in V1 due to right ventricular hypertrophy*

- avoid if possible

    contacts in flu season

    going out   cold

               damp

               fogs

    sedatives, hypnotics

    inessential operations involving anaesthetics

- reduce obesity

    increases respiratory demands

    reduces respiratory efficiency

- combat depression – an optimistic outlook is better than psychotropic drugs

- regular medical supervision is of value

    to detect early and treat acute exacerbations

    to detect and treat cor pulmonale

    to encourage and support

- education of the family and the patient will be very valuable on

    nature of chronic bronchitis

    dangers of continued smoking

    chronic condition – treatment needs to be continuous

    other factors producing exacerbations

    types of treatment available

specific treatment

infection

- *H. influenzae* and *S. pneumoniae* most frequent
- start broad spectrum antibiotic promptly
- if uncontrolled in 5 days try co-trimoxazole (Septrin)
- if still uncontrolled examine sputum

small airway obstruction

- may be

    reversible

        mucosal oedema/inflammation

        mucus obstruction

        bronchospasm

    irreversible

        loss of elasticity (emphysema)

        fibrosis and stenosis

- always try *antibiotics* – start promptly

- deep breathing and chest tapping by relatives may help to move mucus

- *cough medicines*

    expectorants – supposed to encourage sputum

    linctuses – to suppress cough

    little scientific evidence for either effect,

    but useful as placebos

    use linctus to suppress cough when sleep is constantly disturbed by a dry irritant cough – codeine and pholcodine are effective but are constipating

    steam inhalations are helpful in loosening sputum

- *bronchodilators* are always worth a trial in chronic bronchitis since bronchospasm is often present

aerosols – more effective than oral preparations

ß-stimulants
   salbutamol (Ventolin)
   terbutaline (Bricanyl)
   rimiterol (Pulmadil)
   fenoterol (Berotec)

Sympathomimetic
   orciprenaline (Alupent)
   isoprenaline (Medihaler) – dangerous if used excessively

Anticholingergic
   ipratropium (Atrovent)

---

oral preparations

---

aminophylline (Phyllocontin)	100–300 mg p.r.n.
choline theophyllinate (Choledyl)	200 mg t.d.s.
proxyphylline (Thean)	300 mg t.d.s
	600 mg at night
theophylline (Nuelin)	60–200 mg t.d.s.

---

steroids – should be tried if small airway obstruction is resistant to other treatment
   may relieve bronchospasm
   may reduce mucosal oedema
aerosol
   beclomethasone (Becotide, Becloforte)
   betamethasone (Bextasol)
tablets of prednisolone
   10 mg t.d.s. to start
   reduce by 5 mg each day

anoxaemia

- domiciliary oxygen valuable
- concentration no more than 24–28% otherwise the necessary anoxic stimulus to the respiratory centre may be diminished and respiratory failure follow

heart failure

- loop diuretic is mainstay of treatment
    - frusemide (Lasix) 40–120 mg/day
    - ethacrynic acid (Edecrin) 50–300 mg/day
    - bumetanide (Burinex) 1–4 mg/day
- watch out for hypokalaemia (K < 3.5 mmol/1)
    - excessive fatigue
    - cardiac arrhythmia – especially on digoxin
- treat hypokalaemia
    - K supplements – least effective
    - spironolactone (Aldactone)
    - K-retaining diuretic best
        - triamterene (Dytac) 150–250 mg/day
        - amiloride (Midamor) 5–10 mg/day
- digoxin
    - very little value if sinus rhythm
    - always use if atrial fibrillation
    - watch out for arrhythmia
        - undue bradycardia
        - ventricular ectopics
        - ventricular tachycardia
        - atrial tachycardia with a–v block
- salt restriction useful
    - no salt added at table → 3–5 g/day
    - no salt in cooking → 1 g/day

rehabilitation

- retraining

  government retraining courses available

  likelihood of return to suitable gainful employment in severely handicapped chronic bronchitic is remote; demoralization and depression frequent as a result

- exercise

  may be useful in less-disabled

  programme of progressive exercise may increase exercise tolerance

  oxygen before, during and after the exercise may help

- breathing exercises (**phys**iotherapy) may be helpful in preventing stagnation of sputum in bronchioles

social services

home nurses help

- bathing, washing
- check drugs
- instruct re oxygen administration
- breathing exercises/postural drainage
- provide aids – stick, commode etc
- check chiropody needs
- arrange home modifications

social service worker may help

- counselling on finance
- advice on allowances   attendance

  mobility

  heating

- arrange home helps
- arrange meals on wheels
- arrange day centre attendance
- arrange 'night-sitters' if necessary
- investigate rehousing

Useful practical points

- don't accept haemoptysis as a symptom of chronic bronchitis until other causes, especially bronchial carcinoma, have been excluded – bronchoscopy is mandatory
- paroxysmal nocturnal dyspnoea may occur in chronic bronchitis and may be related to the condition or due to coexistent left ventricular failure – the symptoms, signs and response to bronchodilators will help to distinguish the two conditions
- antibiotic treatment of acute exacerbations should be empirical and not dependent on bacteriological examination of the sputum
- it is a good idea to provide the patient with a supply of a broad-spectrum antibiotic (ampicillin, tetracycline) to use at his own discretion if his sputum becomes green or yellow
- avoid hypnotics in severe cases of chronic bronchitis – they may produce respiratory failure
- stopping smoking is the most important single factor in preventing deterioration in chronic bronchitis

6   # CATARRHAL CHILDREN

WHAT IS IT?

- the '*catarrhal child syndrome*' is the most prevalent syndrome in childhood throughout the world

- although it is a collection of apparently distinct clinical conditions, probably it is a single pathological entity

- *components*

    coughs, colds, catarrh

    acute throat infections

    acute otitis media and glue ear

    acute chest infections

- *a single entity because*

    similar age prevalence

    similar aetiology

    similar immunology

    similar natural history

    similar therapeutic frustrations and dilemmas

causes

it is difficult to relate causal agents to clinical presentation, because

    the same organism (bacterial/viral) can produce different clinical condition

    the same clinical condition can be produced by a number of different organisms

coughs, colds and catarrh

- in many no causal pathogen can be isolated and it may be that these are not infections but forms of reactive hypersensitivity to external non-pathogenic irritants or allergens

- where a pathogen is isolated it is usually a virus such as

  rhinovirus

  adenovirus

  enterovirus

  respiratory syncytial virus (RSV)

  parainfluenza virus

  influenza

  laryngotracheobronchitis (croup) often caused by RSV and parainfluenza

  acute epiglottitis caused by *Haemophilus influenzae* bacteria

acute throat infection

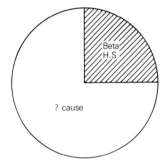

- in only one quarter are ß-haemolytic streptococci isolated
- some may be due to the viruses noted
- in many no pathogen isolated

acute otitis media

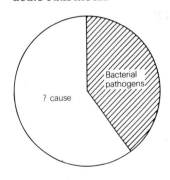

- bacterial pathogens in about one third to one half

  H. influenzae

  Streptococcus pneumoniae

  ß-haemolytic streptococcus

- viruses are not often isolated

acute chest infections

- *infants*

  RSV
  parainfluenzae } viruses

  Streptococcus pneumoniae
  Haemophilus influenzae
  ß-haemolytic streptococci
  staphylococci } bacteria

- *older children*

  Streptococcus pneumoniae
  Haemophilus influenzae
  Mycoplasma pneumoniae } bacteria

  influenza
  adenovirus } viruses

clinical

coughs, colds and catarrh

- Recurrent upper respiratory infection predominantly with blocked, running noses and cough

acute throat infections

- red fauces
- swollen red tonsils
- exudate
- cervical glands +
- *note*   croup
  epiglottitis

acute otitis media

- earache/red drum
- deafness
- discharge

acute chest infections

- acute wheezy chest (bronchitis/ bronchopneumonia)
- localized crackles (pneumonia/pneumonitis)
- generalized crackles (bronchiolitis/ pneumonia)

114

infants

- do not complain of local symptoms, earache or sore throat and may present as acute febrile illness with vague tummy ache

WHO GETS IT WHEN?

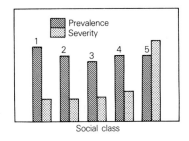

- *all children* suffer at some time
- equal prevalence throughout social classes – but more severe and complications in lower social classes

age prevalence

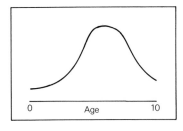

- characteristic age prevalence for all components of syndrome
- onset → peak → decline
- peak prevalence age 4–8 years
- tendency for natural remission after age 8 years

frequency

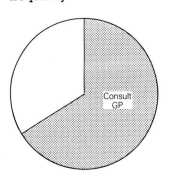

- in any year, two thirds of all children (0–10) consult GP for the syndrome – 300 children per 2500 practice (each with three to four consultations)

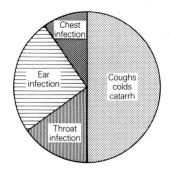

coughs, cold, catarrh	50%
acute throat infections	15%
acute otitis media	25%
acute chest infections	10%
	100%

general practice

general practice 2500 persons (300 children under 10 years):

Annual numbers of children consulting

coughs, colds, catarrh	160
acute throat infection	15
acute otitis media	40
acute chest infections	12

district general hospital

DGH for 250 000 population

For catarrhal children

Annual OPD referrals	
Paediatrician	500
ENT	600

Annual admissions	
Paediatrician	250
ENT	
T & A	250
Ears etc	200

WHAT HAPPENS?

onset → peak → remission

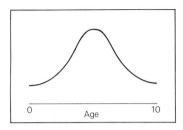

- this is an almost inevitable syndrome of childhood
- it is a 'normal abnormality' which is self-limiting
- probable explanation is that it represents an immunological reaction to 'social mixing' and reactions in respiratory tract to infections and irritants by an immature immune system

acute throat infections

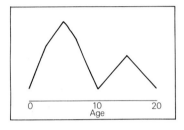

- in some children there is recurrence in the teens – at the glandular fever age period, perhaps another immunological process
- tonsillectomy probably necessary in 5%

acute otitis media

- 'glue ear' in about 20% but most resolve in time
- grommets – how many really necessary?
- chronic discharge rare
- permanent hearing loss of some degree (mostly slight) in 10%

acute chest infections

- acute wheezy chests in children – only 5% become adult asthmatics
- few may become 'chronic bronchitics' in adult life (possibly vulnerable respiratory tract)

WHAT TO DO?

issues

- a 'normal abnormality'
- benign but causes much distress, suffering and anxiety during periods of activity
- uncertain causes
- uncertainties on effective management

- tendency to 'natural cure'
- treatments
    palliatives
    specific
        antibiotics?
        surgery?

diagnosis

- *clinical* examination and assessment are most useful
- bacteriology
    throat swabs – limited value
        only one quarter of acute throat infections grow ß-haemolytic streptococci
- blood
    only useful in excluding glandular fever
    immune deficiency syndromes very rare
- chest X-rays
    only in atypical chest infections
- audiometry
    very useful in children over 6 (cooperation difficult under this age)
    if deafness found, follow-up until hearing returns to normal, and if delayed refer to specialist
- respiratory function
    peak flow meter in recurrent wheezers

differential diagnosis

- *allergic nose* (vasomotor rhinitis) – recurring 'colds' often seasonal or early morning, FH+, nose rubbing
- *asthma* – recurring wheezy chests unrelated to infections, FH+
- *glandular fever* – usually in teenagers but can occur in younger children; tonsillitis+ with glands + and no response to antibiotics

- *fibrocystic disease* – recurring severe chest infections, infected (bacterial) sputum, slow physical development, nasal polypi, diarrhoea
- *immune deficiency* – recurring severe chest infections

TREATMENT

the most important part in good management is to spend time in explaining the nature, inevitability, normality, course and outcomes – to parents – and to be prepared for care and support over a few years

relief

- earache, sore throat

    analgesics – paracetamol/aspirin
- cough

    hot drinks

    simple linctus
- nasal obstruction
    vasoconstrictor nose drops (of uncertain value)

antibiotics

- majority of infections are not caused by pathogenic bacteria
- uncertain case for using antibiotics in all cases of ear, throat and chest infections
- most will recover without antibiotics
- indications for antibiotics

    degree of illness

    severity of symptoms

    presenting signs

    previous history

    views and philosophy of physician

- choice

    ampicillin

    amoxycillin

    trimethoprim

    co-trimoxazole

    erythromycin

    flucloxacillin

    penicillin for acute strep. throats

surgery

- *tonsillectomy*

    for repeated tonsillitis – probably in only 5–10% of children

- *adenoidectomy*

    for recurring otitis media

    for persistent deafness

    for ear discharge

    for nasal obstruction

- *grommets* and tympanotomy/aspiration

    for persistent deafness

    for fluid in middle ear

- *myringotomy*

    rarely indicated in acute otitis media

Useful practical points

- inevitable 'normal abnormality' of childhood
- syndrome a collection of parts – nose, throat, ears and chest infections
- peak prevalence at 4–8 years followed by natural remission
- management must always bear in mind the likelihood of full spontaneous recovery
- antibiotics – should be used with selective discrimination
- surgery – should be used with selective discrimination too

7

GLANDULAR FEVER (INFECTIOUS MONONUCLEOSIS)

WHAT IS IT?

- infectious mononucleosis (IM) is now considered to be an infection caused by the Epstein–Barr virus (EBV). The virus infects B-lymphocytes with a reactive response by T-lymphocytes that destroy EBV
- EB virus is excreted in oropharyngeal secretions during the infection and for several months afterwards
- similar clinical syndromes result from infections by cytomegalovirus and in toxoplasmosis
- predominantly a condition of teenagers and young adults and particularly those in relatively closed communities as universities and military establishments

clinical features (see Figure 7.1)

- gradual onset with persistent symptoms
- sore throat with tonsillitis
- enlarged and tender lymph glands, prominent in neck, but generalized
- fever and general malaise
- splenomegaly
- hepatitis – clinical/biochemical
- skin rash – especially after ampicillin

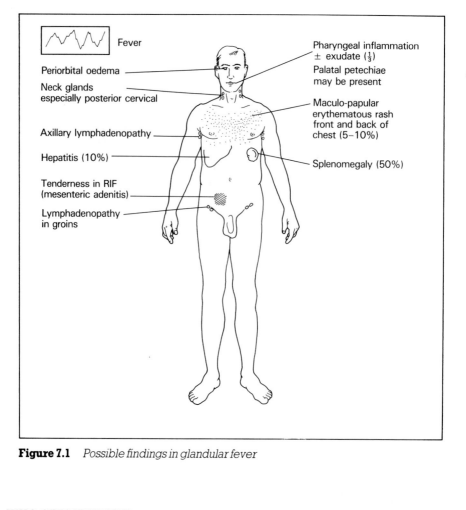

Figure 7.1 *Possible findings in glandular fever*

WHO GETS IT WHEN?

frequency

- annual incidence is about two per 1000 (five in practice of 2500), but probably higher in universities

general practice

general practice with 2500 persons

Annual new cases	
incidence	5
(mild	3)
(moderate	2)
(severe	<1)

district general hospital	DGH with 250 000 population
	Annual new cases glandular fever admitted 25

age – sex prevalence

- peak at 15–25 (can occur at any age but exceptional in infancy and old age – beware of making diagnosis of IM then)
- M = F

social class

- probably affects classes equally but because more upper classes attend universities it is believed to affect upper social class
- subclinical infection common in children from poor homes

seasonal

- peak prevalence in winter and autumn

infectivity

- although labelled as 'infectious', in normal practice IM occurs *sporadically* and *not* epidemically
- incubation period may be 2–3 weeks
- in universities *epidemics* may occur or perhaps it is *endemic*
- believed to be spread by droplets and kissing (hence 'kissing disease')
- antibodies to EBV are widespread in persons who have never had clinical IM – hence *subclinical infection* is common

WHAT HAPPENS?

course

- resolution of acute symptoms over 2–3 weeks
- lethargy and depression may *persist* over weeks or months, though how much of this is due to real effects of virus infection, and what the mechanism is, remain unknown

- attacks vary in *severity: from* mild and
  subclinical cases *to* very severe illness with
  throat infection + +, high fever and toxaemia
- following IM, teenagers may suffer from
  recurring acute tonsillitis that requires
  tonsillectomy
- *second attacks* are unusual but can occur[1]

family cases

- there are families where all the children suffer
  from IM when they reach teenage – these are
  not cross-infections but probably an
  immunological state of hypersensitivity to
  EBV[1]

lymphoma

- an apparent case of IM may rarely progress to
  a lymphoma[1]

complications (see Figure 7.2)

common

- skin rash

    erythematous macules

    often on 5th day of infection

    may be precipitated by antibiotic
    especially ampicillin

- severe pharyngeal inflammation and
  swelling
- post-infective depression

uncommon

- cardiac   myocarditis (may be fatal)
                  pericarditis
- neurological
    encephalitis   Guillain–Barré syndrome
                         cranial nerve palsies
                         transverse myelitis

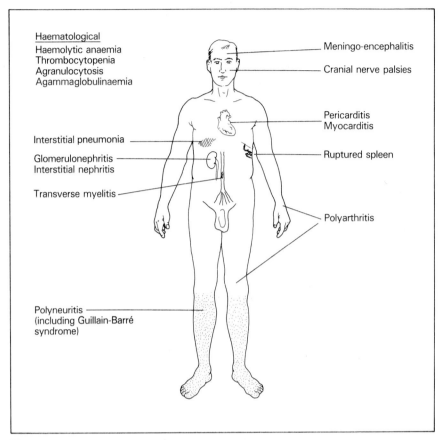

Figure 7.2 *Possible complications of glandular fever*

- renal
    glomerulonephritis
    interstitial nephritis
- lungs – interstitial pneumonia
- polyarthritis
- haematological
    haemolytic anaemia
    thrombocytopenia
    agranulocytosis
    agammaglobulinaemia
- splenic rupture with trauma

WHAT TO DO?

issues
- a condition of teenagers/young adults
- believed to be caused by EBV but of low infectivity – probably much subclinical infection
- benign course but complications do occur
- satisfying diagnosis (for doctor) but no specific therapy

diagnosis
- think of IM in any sore throat in teenager that persists for longer than 1–2 weeks
- diagnosis of IM only on confirmation by blood tests

blood
- total lymphocyte/monocyte count 50–60%
- atypical mononuclear lymphocytes (20% or more)
- positive Paul–Bunnell test: titres of heterophil antibodies start rising 4th 7th day of the illness
- positive Monospot screening test for heterophil antibodies
- 'positives' appear early in infection (50–80% in first 10 days) and may persist for 3 months
- if first Paul–Bunnell negative – repeat
- 10% of adults with IM, and even more children, do not produce heterophil antibodies at any time and so the Paul–Bunnell and Monospot tests remain persistently negative

virology
- EBV – specific IgM indicates current primary infection
- EBV IgG indicates past infection

differential diagnosis

acute throat infection

- types

  streptococcal
  diphtheria
  viral

  distinguish by   sudden onset

                         rapid recovery

                         no lymphocytosis

                         negative Monospot/Paul–Bunnell

                         culture from throat swab

rubella

- lymphocytes may be atypical and so suggest IM
- distinguish by   sudden onset

                         short duration

                         lack of systemic upset
- negative Monospot/Paul–Bunnell

leukaemia

- distinguish by   progressive deterioration

                         bleeding frequent

                         blood picture

                         bone marrow examination

cytomegalovirus

- may show atypical lymphocytes
- distinguish by increase in cytomegalovirus complement-fixing titres

toxoplasmosis

- distinguish by rise in toxoplasma titres

malignancy

- high titres of antibodies to EB virus found in

  Burkitt's lymphoma

  retropharyngeal carcinoma

  other lymphoproliferative conditions in patients with congenital or acquired immune-deficiency states, e.g. AIDS

- role of EB virus unclear
- could be opportunist infection
- could be contributory causal factor
- distinguish by gland/growth biopsy

infective hepatitis

- occasionally shows atypical lymphocytes
- distinguish by measurement of hepatitis A, B and non-A, non-B virus antigens and antibodies

TREATMENT

- no specific treatment against EB virus
- secondary streptococcal pharyngitis may occur

  treat with penicillin or erythromycin

  avoid ampicillin and other semisynthetic penicillins (e.g. amoxycillin) because of the risk of rash

- metronidazole may be helpful in treating non-streptococcal throat infection in IM
- indication for steroid treatment

  severe pharyngeal infection

  neurological complications

  hepatitis

  intestitial pneumonia

  laryngeal obstruction

  haemolytic anaemia

  severe thrombocytopenic purpura

- dose of steroids

  80 mg daily first day

  45 mg daily 2 days

  30 mg daily 2 days

  15 mg daily for last 2 days

- convalescent phase – avoid athletic activities if splenomegaly is present because of the risk of trauma and rupture

Useful practical points

- think of IM in teenager with persisting sore throat with cervical glands
- think of IM (subclinical) if persisting malaise, lethargy and depression in teenager
- benign and self-limiting
- low infectivity – epidemics are unusual
- no specific therapy
- beware of ampicillin/amoxycillin in sore throats – cause rashes in IM
- recurrences do occur
- there are families where all siblings suffer IM on reaching vulnerable age
- if the clinical picture suggests glandular fever and the Paul–Bunnell test is persistently negative, always consider cytomegalic virus and toxoplasmosis

8   PEPTIC ULCERS

WHAT ARE THEY?

- symptom complexes (syndromes) with objective evidence of gastric/duodenal ulceration (G.U./D.U.) by radiology and/or endoscopy
- D.U. : G.U. is 4 : 1

symptoms

- *pain* occurs in 80% of patients
- the *typical features* of the pain are:

    epigastric

    gnawing or burning

    related to food

    remissions and relapses

    relieved by alkalis

- there are some *differentiating features* between the pain of gastric and duodenal ulcers but there is considerable overlap

	Gastric ulcer	Duodenal ulcer
Relation to meals	½ – 2 h after	just before
Effect of food	worse	better
Vomiting	common	rare (unless stenosis)
Nocturnal pain	rare	common
Penetration to back	very rare	frequent

- Crean's study (1984) showed the similarity of symptoms between gastric and duodenal ulcer

	D.U. (%)	G.U. (%)
Epigastric pain	74	65
Episodic	86	69
Relief from antacids	65	66
Night pain	40	31
F.H.	40	50

Data: ref. 16

- ulcer pain can occur in sites other than the epigastrium

  elsewhere in abdomen

  interscapular area (penetrating D.U.)

  retrosternal

- 'non-ulcer dyspepsia' – typical ulcer symptoms may occur with no objective evidence of peptic ulcer
- severity of ulcer pain is no guide to prognosis – a large ulcer can be painless
- ulcer symptoms de novo may be associated with gastric cancer

signs

- the only sign of uncomplicated peptic ulcer is epigastric tenderness
- if pyloric stenosis is present there may be:

  upper abdominal distension

  visible peristaltic waves

  succussion splash on palpation

- if there is significant weight loss suspect gastric carcinoma

causes
the causation of peptic ulcer is uncertain but there are a number of relevant factors

constitutional diathesis in D.U.

- blood group O more frequent
- non-secretion of blood group antigens in the saliva more frequent
- family history – 40% of D.U. patients have at least one other family member affected
- 50% chance of concordant ulcer in identical twins – 14% in dizygotic twins
- HLA-B5 antigen more frequent

geographical

- D.U. commoner in Scotland and north of England than in the south of Britain
- G.U. commoner in north Wales and south-east England.
- D.U. commoner in south India than in the north of India and five times commoner than G.U.
- G.U. three times more frequent than D.U. in Japan

cigarette smoking

- small but definite increase in smokers
- mortality from ulcer is higher in smokers
- slower healing of ulcers on treatment in smokers

social class

- more frequent in poorer people in Western countries
- suggested more frequent in stressful occupations – no supporting evidence
- mortality higher in unskilled workers

hormonal influences

- peptic ulcer uncommon in pregnancy
- oestrogens can promote healing of ulcer

associated diseases

- higher incidence than expected in patients with

  chronic bronchitis

  ischaemic heart disease

  pulmonary tuberculosis (in G.U.)

  chronic renal failure (in D.U.)

- increased incidence also in

  hyperparathyroidism

  polycythaemia vera

drugs

- three groups of drugs are relevant

  aspirin

  non-steroidal anti-inflammatory drugs

  steroids

- the evidence of correlation is, however, weak

WHO GETS IT AND WHEN?

age prevalence (annual consulting rates)

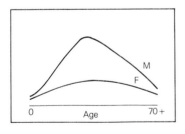

- *D.U.* M > F

  peak at 35–55

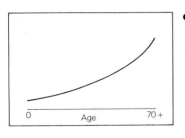

- *G.U.* M = F

  rise with age

age at diagnosis

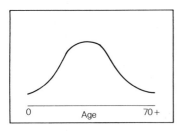

- *D.U.* peak onset at 20–40

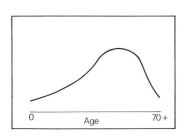

- *G.U.* peak onset at 40–60

frequency

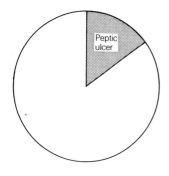

- a European/American has up to one in seven chance of suffering from a peptic ulcer during a lifetime[17,18]:

  male 10–15%

  female 8–10%

general practice

general practice with 2500 persons : peptic ulcers:

Annual new cases diagnosed (incidence)	5–10 (decreasing)
Annual patients consulting (prevalence)	35
Persons with past and present history of peptic ulcers	100

Data : ref. 1

district general hospital	DGH with 250 000 population: peptic ulcers:	
	Annual admissions	500
	Endoscopies (if active units)	up to 1000

WHAT HAPPENS?

mortality

- peptic ulcers cause symptoms but not death – but deaths do occur from *complications*

    bleeding

    perforation

natural history : course and outcome

- there is a natural tendency for symptoms to remit spontaneously and for ulcers to heal

    spontaneous healing of D.U. and G.U.

    40% healed in 4 weeks

    60% healed in 6 weeks

    80% healed in 8 weeks

recurrences

- *recurrences are frequent*

    in 80% symptoms recur in 12 months

- *eventually* majority will cease to suffer symptoms

    one quarter suffer one attack only, followed by no recurrence

    one half suffer recurring bouts controlled with medication (antacids)

    one quarter suffer severe and persistent symptoms[19]

periods of activity

- *periods of activity* of symptoms are likely for 10–15 years followed by remission, often complete

surgery

- over 5 to 10 years:

    G.U. – 1 in 4 may come to operation

    D.U. – 1 in 7 may come to operation (*see* trends on pages 149–150)

follow-up

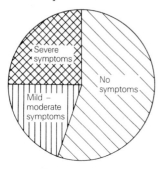

- *duodenal ulcers*[1,20]

    55% : *no symptoms*

    20% : *mild–moderate symptoms*

    25% : *severe symptoms*

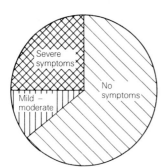

- *gastric ulcers*[1]

    64% : *no symptoms*

    11% : *mild–moderate symptoms*

    25% : *severe symptoms*

complications

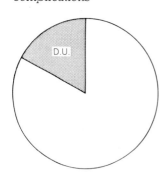

- *haemorrhage*

    bleeding   D.U. 17%

    G.U. 10%

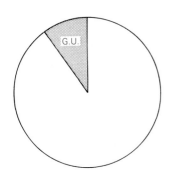

recurrent bleeds 25–30% [17]

- *surgery* for 25%
- *perforation* D.U. 3%

  G.U. 1% (associated with bleed – 10%)

(these observations *before* availability of H_2–receptor antagonists – now results are much better)

mortality from complications

- *bleeding and age* [17]

  < 60 – 5% mortality

  60–79 – 10% mortality

  over 80 – 25% mortality

- *perforation* [17]

  D.U. 5–15%

  G.U. 10–40%

WHAT TO DO?

diagnosis

- since symptoms are unreliable in either diagnosing peptic ulcer or distinguishing accurately between gastric and duodenal ulcer, the diagnosis must be made by either barium meal or endoscopy
- the advantages and disadvantages of barium meal and endoscopy are shown in the table

	Barium meal	Endoscopy
Advantages	• simple • inexpensive • widely available • little discomfort	• accurate • reliable • distinguishes benign and malignant ulcers • can take biopsy • can assess healing • can control bleeding
Disadvantages	• may miss ulcer (10–30%) • poor differentiation between benign and malignant	• not readily available • uncomfortable • complications – perforated oesophagus, burst recent perforation, burst recently healed ulcer

barium meal changes

- gastric ulcer (benign) (Figure 8.1)
    clean niche of barium

    undercut surrounding mucosa

    usually lesser curve
- gastric ulcer (malignant) (Figure 8.2)
    flat or irregular erosion

    surrounding mucosal oedema

    greater curve or antrum

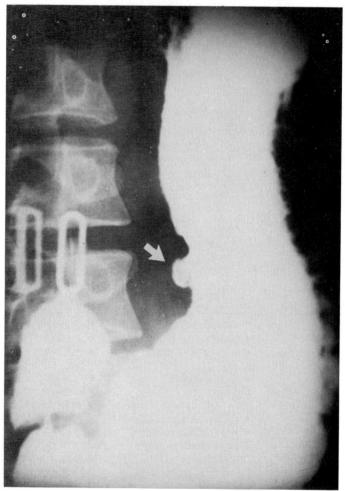

Figure 8.1 *Barium meal showing niche on lesser curve (arrowed) due to a benign gastric ulcer*

PEPTIC ULCERS

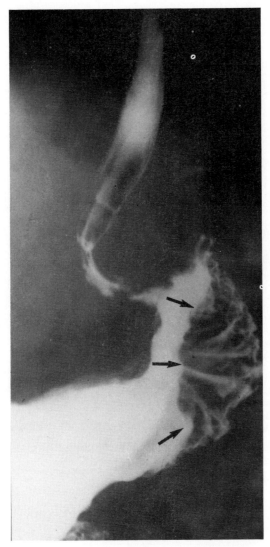

Figure 8.2 *Barium meal showing filling defect in the fundus of the stomach (arrowed) due to carcinoma*

- duodenal ulcer (Figure 8.3)

  scarred duodenal cap

  very difficult to see ulcer

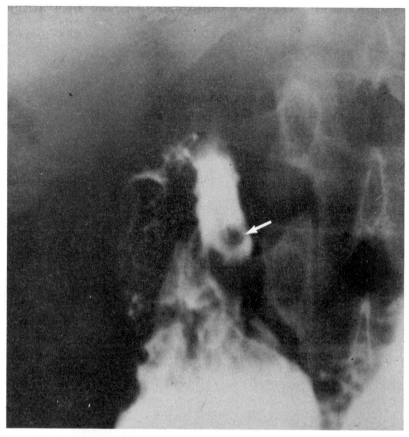

Figure 8.3 *Barium meal showing filling defect in the 1st part of the duodenum due to acute inflammatory change in a duodenal ulcer*

indications for endoscopy

- gastric ulcer

    to exclude malignancy

    to establish initial diagnosis prior to treatment

    to assess healing

- duodenal ulcer – prior to surgery

- to diagnose and control gastroduodenal bleed

- suggestive symptoms but equivocal barium meal

- equivocal barium meal and no response to treatment

measurement of gastric acidity – no value in the routine diagnosis of peptic ulcer. Indications

- recurrent ulcer after surgery
- diagnosis of Zollinger–Ellison syndrome

TREATMENT

with *no treatment* most ulcers apparently heal, many recur episodically and eventually many cease to suffer symptoms

aims of treatment

- relief of symptoms
- healing of the ulcer
- prevention of recurrence
- prevention of complications

medical treatment

medical treatment can relieve pain and heal the ulcer but cannot prevent reoccurrence or complications

basis of medical treatment

- general measures
- symptomatic treatment
- specific treatment

general measures

- bed rest
- stop smoking – more effective in G.U.
- diet

  can relieve symptoms

  no value in healing ulcer
- avoid gastric irritants

  aspirin

  other anti-inflammatory drugs

  steroids

- there is no good evidence that sedation, or restriction of tea, coffee or alcohol has any value

symptomatic treatment

- relief of pain is achieved by *antacids* – the neutralizing capacity is irrelevant since small doses will relieve pain as effectively as large doses

water-soluble	sodium bicarbonate
	calcium carbonate
water-insoluble	aluminium salts
	magnesium salts

- side-effects of antacids

  magnesium trisilicate $\rightarrow$ diarrhoea

  aluminium hydroxide $\rightarrow$ constipation

  sodium bicarbonate $\rightarrow$ alkalosis

  calcium carbonate   alkalosis

                         hypercalcaemia

                         renal failure

  impaired drug absorption, e.g. tetracycline, chlorpromazine, can occur with all Ca, Al or Mg-containing antacids

- there are many compound proprietary antacid preparations but there is no evidence that they are any more effective than simple preparations

- *anticholinergic* drugs (e.g. Pro-Banthine, Kolanticon) – there is little place for these drugs in treating peptic ulcer because of their limited effectiveness in the standard dose and because of their side-effects, especially in the elderly:

  glaucoma

  blurring of vision

  dry mouth

  urinary retention

  constipation

specific treatment

there are four treatments which can heal ulcers

- H$_2$-receptor blockers

    cimetidine (Tagamet)

    ranitidine (Zantac)

- carbenoxolone (Biogastrone)
- colloidal bismuthate (De-Nol)
- high-dose antacids

H$_2$-receptor blockers – 50% of ulcers heal within 3 weeks and 90% within 6 weeks

    dose

        cimetidine – 200 mg t.d.s.

                     400 mg at night   } 4 weeks

                     400 mg at night –

                     maintenance

        ranitidine – 150 mg b.d. for 4 weeks

                     150 mg at night –

                     maintenance

Recent work suggests that cimetidine in a dose of 400 mg b.d. may be as effective in healing ulcers as the standard larger dose

maintenance treatment – because of the high rate of relapse when the H$_2$-blocker is stopped, maintenance treatment is required: a 3-month course can be tried and if there are further relapses these can be treated by further short courses, by a prolonged course or probably best by surgery since the hazards of prolonged treatment with H$_2$-blockers are not known, especially the risk of gastric carcinoma

side-effects of cimetidine

    gynaecomastia

    confusion especially elderly

    diarrhoea

    interferes with other drugs

        phenytoin

        warfarin

ranitidine does not have similar side-effects

carbenoxolone – this is as effective as cimetidine in promoting healing of gastric ulcer but may be less effective in duodenal ulcer, though a special preparation is available (Duogastrone)

dose – 50–100 mg t.d.s. for 4–6 weeks

side-effects – these are relevant especially to the elderly, and the drug is therefore contraindicated in these patients

salt/water retention ⌐oedema

hypertension

heart failure

hypokalaemia – muscle weakness

colloidal bismuthate – this too is as effective as cimetidine and there is some evidence that relapse of ulcer is less frequent

dose – 5 ml (120 mg) four times daily for 4–6 weeks – the taste is unpleasant

side-effects

blackens teeth and tongue

blackens stool – may confuse with melaena

interferes with tetracyclines

high-dose antacids – this involves taking up to 200–300 ml aluminium hydroxide daily and is impracticable

surgery

15% of D.U. are resistant to H_2-antagonists, likely to be

young onset

long history

FH+

indications for surgical treatment of peptic ulcer

- failure to heal after adequate medical treatment

- complications

    uncontrollable bleeding

    perforation

    stenosis

        pyloric ulcer

        hourglass stomach

- recurrent gastric ulcer
- recurrent ulcer after previous surgery
- unacceptable disruption of work/leisure

    suspicion of malignancy in a gastric ulcer is no longer an indication for surgery since the diagnosis can be established by gastroscopy

types of surgery

- *Billroth 1* – operation of choice for gastric ulcer (Figure 8.4)

    advantage – preserves continuity of GI tract

    disadvantage – dumping and biliary reflux

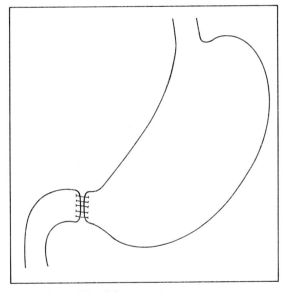

Figure 8.4   *Billroth 1 gastrectomy*

- vagotomy – for duodenal ulcer (Figure 8.5)

  truncal (+ pyloroplasty)

advantages	easy to do
	possible in poor risks and in emergencies
disadvantages	high recurrence rate
	diarrhoea
	dumping
	biliary reflux

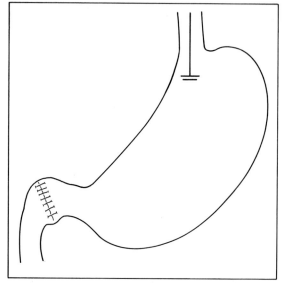

Figure 8.5   *Truncal vagotomy + pyloroplasty*

proximal (selective) – preserves nerve supply to antrum and pylorus (Figure 8.6)

advantages	safest (gut not opened)
	minimizes after-effects
	dumping
	biliary reflux
	diarrhoea
disadvantages	
	technically difficult
	high recurrence rate

PEPTIC ULCERS

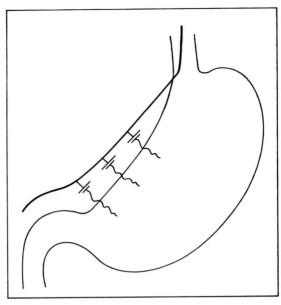

Figure 8.6   *Proximal vagotomy*

adverse after-effects of surgery   mechanical
- vomiting
- dumping
- diarrhoea

nutritional
- iron deficiency anaemia
- B_{12} deficiency
- osteomalacia
- osteoporosis

results   results after surgery are good so that surgery should not be delayed if indicated[21]:

vagotomy and antrectomy – 99% healing

proximal gastric vagotomy – 91% healing

management of complications of peptic ulcer

bleeding
- hospital admission
- assess circulatory state – pulse and BP
- blood transfusion if
    Hb < 10 g/dl
    clinical shock
    excessive visible blood loss
- early endoscopy or barium examination
- most settle within 4 days
- recurrent bleeding → surgery

factors increasing mortality
- > 40 years old
- chronic ulcer
- rebleeding

perforation
- confirmation by X-ray – gas under diaphragm in 80%
- management
    treat for shock
    simple closure if in poor condition
    closure + definitive operation best
        G.U. → partial gastrectomy
        D.U. → vagotomy + pyloroplasty
- if unfit for operation treat conservatively
    intravenous fluids
    regular gastric aspiration
    parenteral nutrition
    systemic antibiotics

mortality 5% – elderly fare worse

outlet stenosis

- diagnosis

    long history of ulcer

    large vomit containing food

    wasting and dehydration

    visible peristalsis

    succussion splash

- investigation

    gastric aspiration – large volume

    barium meal/endoscopy

- treatment

    pyloric stenosis →vagotomy + drainage operation

    duodenal stenosis → vagotomy + Billroth 1

TRENDS

- *hospital admissions* (UK) (1958–77)

    for D.U. reduced by 30%

    for G.U. reduced by 50%

- *mortality rates* (UK) (1958–77)

    for D.U. reduced by 40%

    for G.U. reduced by 40%

- *peptic ulcers* (USA) (1965–80)

    mortality – reduced by two thirds

    first diagnosis – reduced by one third

    surgical operations (vagotomy and partial gastrectomy) – reduced by 44% [17]

- the decline in gastric surgery has occurred without corresponding falls for other abdominal operations[23]

Abdominal surgical operations per 10 000 in USA

	1970	1978
All	122	132
Vagotomy and PG	6	3
Appendicectomy	16	14
Cholecystectomy	18	20
Hernia	25	24

- the falls in gastric surgery are likely because of H_2-antagonists

---

Useful practical points

- although still common, the prevalence of peptic ulcers has fallen in past decade – probably a natural event, but may have been helped by H_2-antagonists
- peptic ulcers still are potentially dangerous from their complications, i.e. bleeding and perforation
- there is a strong natural tendency for peptic ulcers to heal, they should be allowed the opportunity
- H_2-antagonists are the most effective known antacid drugs, but they should be used with care and discrimination

---

9   GALLSTONES

WHAT ARE THEY?

- gallstones are formed from constituents of bile and are found most often in the gallbladder
- *types of gallstones* – three types

> pigment stones – contain bilirubin and Ca salts – small black multiple
>
> cholesterol stones – contain > 95% cholesterol – may be
>
>   solitary large oval
>
>   multiple small yellow
>
>   two large stones indenting
>
> mixed stones – contain alternating layers cholesterol, bile pigment, Ca salts

pathogenesis

- three basic factors involved
  - stasis in biliary tract
  - infection
  - alterations in bile
- *pigment stones* – excessive bilirubin production due to:
  - chronic haemolytic anaemia
    - congenital spherocytosis
    - thalassaemia
    - sickle cell anaemia
  - cirrhosis

- *cholesterol stones*

  high concentration of cholesterol in bile relative to bile salts and phospholipids → precipitation

  gallstone patients have increased hepatic cholesterol synthesis and reduced bile salt synthesis

predisposing conditions

the traditional stereotype patient who develops gallbladder disease is still relevant in diagnosis today

  female

  fair

  fat

  forty

  fertile

other relevant factors

- obesity
- diet – high fat/low roughage
- oestrogens   contraceptive pill

        menopausal treatment

        high parity in women
- clofibrate treatment
- ileal resection, e.g. in Crohn's disease
- gallstones have increased in prevalence in Western societies over past 50 years
- operations for gallstones have also increased: 45 000 annually in UK; 250 000 annually in USA. Cholecystectomy now is the commonest elective operation in the Western world

WHO GETS THEM WHEN?

- true prevalence of gallstones is difficult to measure because many are 'silent' and do not cause symptoms

autopsies

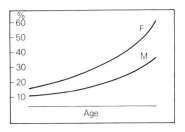

- autopsies show how many of those dying from all causes have gallstones. Data from various sources[24-27] suggests that about 10% of the population have gallstones

    adults (over 30)

    one in three women has gallstones

    one in five men has gallstones

    thus it is likely that in Britain there are 5 million persons with gallstones

	% autopsies with gallstones		
Age	M	F	M : F
30–39	5	12	1 : 2.4
40–49	7	14	1 : 2
50–59	12	25	1 : 2.1
60–69	20	35	1 : 1.8
70–79	28	45	1 : 1.6
80 +	32	59	1 : 1.6
Total over 30	20	33	1 : 1.7
	25		

- autopsy rates of bodies with gallstones have increased ×4 from 1933 to 1970

frequency

general practice

general practice population of 2500 :
gallstones

Annual new cases (incidence)	4
Annual patients consulting (prevalence)	10
Annual cholecystectomies	2
Estimated persons with gallstones (25% of over-30s)	350

- great majority of gallstones are symptomless and are taken to the grave

district general hospital

DGH serving 250 000 people : annual numbers

Admissions for gallbladder disease	250
Cholecystectomies	200
Deaths from cholecystectomy	2
Deaths from cancer of gallbladder	2.5

WHAT HAPPENS?

- *some data* (UK per year)

  5 million with gallstones

  45 000 cholecystectomies[25]

  2000 deaths from gallbladder diseases

  600 deaths from cancer of gallbladder
- it is estimated that 100 cholecystectomies are required to prevent one cancer of gallbladder
- mortality of cholecystectomy is 1%
- it is likely that about one in six of persons with gallstones has a cholecystectomy

- many gallstones are *silent* when detected – i.e. they do not cause symptoms as they lie free in the lumen of the gallbladder
- most gallstones are never detected clinically

natural history

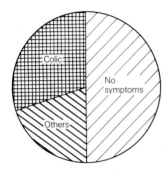

- the likely natural history of gallstones[25,29]

  50% – no symptoms

  33% – colic

  7% – jaundice or pancreatitis

  15% – cholecystectomy

  1% – die from gallbladder disease

  0.05% – develop cancer of gallbladder [29, 25]

morbidity

- *acute impaction in cystic duct*

  biliary colic

  epigastric or right hypochondriac pain

  constant – not colicky

  radiation

  tip of right shoulder

  interscapular area

  pain lasts 10 min – 6 hours

  if the pain lasts over 6 h a complication is likely, e.g. cholecystitis or pancreatitis

  relief when stone disimpacts

- *acute cholecystitis* if stone remains impacted

  diagnosis

  dull central abdominal pain

  may be referred → interscapular area

  abdominal tenderness

  fever

  80% subside spontaneously

complications

    gangrene of gallbladder

    perforation with peritonitis

- *retention of impacted stone in cystic duct*

    recurrent attacks of acute cholecystitis leading to chronic cholangitis with a shrunken fibrosed gallbladder

    hydrops of the gallbladder – painless due to slow distension and excessive mucus secretion

    calcium may collect in the bile ('limey bile') – or in the gallbladder wall ('porcelain gallbladder')

    empyema   persistent pain

                pyrexia

                increasing local signs

                toxaemia

- *passage of stone into common bile duct*

    biliary colic may occur if sudden impaction

    slow occlusion painless (25%)

    obstructive jaundice   dark urine

                          pale stools

    cholangitis

      non-suppurative   fever

                     chills

                     biliary colic

                     jaundice

      suppurative   septic shock

                     liver abscess

    secondary biliary cirrhosis – long term complication if obstruction persists (5 years)

- *other complications of gallstones*

  acute pancreatitis – gallstone found in common bile duct on X-ray in 50%

  severe upper abdominal pain

  tenderness

  rigidity

  shock in severe cases

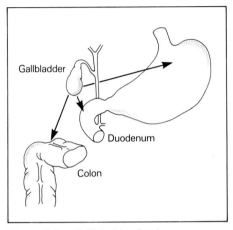

Figure 9.1   *Gallbladder fistulae*

fistula formation – recurrent attacks of acute cholecystitis may lead to fistula formation (Figure 9.1)

duodenum

colon

stomach

rarely with bronchus, ovary, kidney, bladder, uterus

with a large stone (> 2.5 cm diameter) impaction may occur in terminal ileum leading to intestinal obstruction (gallstone ileus)

carcinoma – rare complication

if it does occur 90% of the patients will have chronic cholecystitis

may develop in 50% of patients with 'porcelain' gallbladder (X-ray)

'flatulent dyspepsia'

a symptom complex consisting of

vague epigastric discomfort

belching

flatulence

fatty food intolerance

these symptoms occur with equal frequency in patients with and without gallstones so unlikely to be due to the gallstones

40% will still have same symptoms 5 years after cholecystectomy

WHAT TO DO?

diagnosis

radiology

- *plain X-ray of abdomen* – this is worth doing in all patients. The helpful findings are:

  mixed stones may be seen in up to 30% of cases (Figure 9.2)

  'limey bile'

  'porcelain' gallbladder

  air in biliary tract – fistula

  shadowing due to hydrops or empyema of gallbladder

- *oral cholecystogram*

  identifies 70% of stones

  patient not jaundiced

  gallbladder not seen – suggests obstructed cystic duct

  10% non-visualized gallbladders are seen at second examination

  radiotranslucent stones may be seen (Figure 9.3)

  poorly-functioning gallbladder is not significant since half turn out to be normal

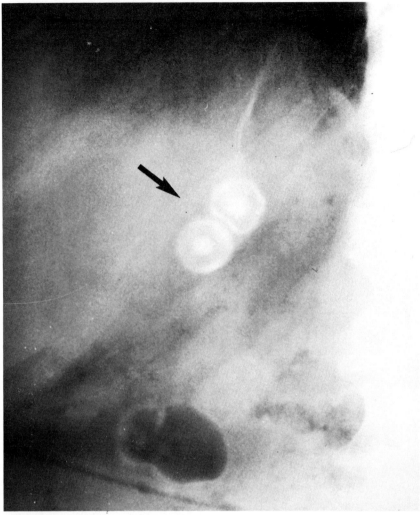

Figure 9.2 *Plain X-ray of gallstones*

- *intravenous cholangiography (IVC)*

    indications

    previous cholecystectomy

    for confirmation of non-visualized
    gallbladder on oral cholecystography

    differential diagnosis of acute abdomen
    to exclude gallstones

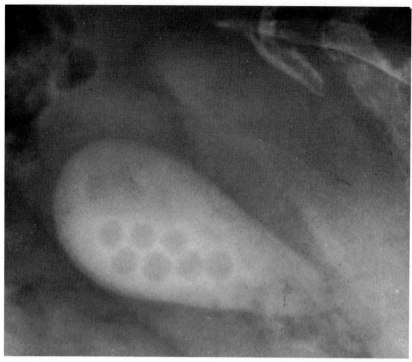

Figure 9.3   *Cholecystogram showing radiotranslucent (cholesterol) stones*

    oral cholecystogram not possible because
    of gastroduodenal disease

    stones suspected in CBD

    liver function tests must be normal

    percutaneous transhepatic cholangiography
    is better if patient is jaundiced

- *ERCP (endoscopic retrograde
  cholangiopancreatography)* – gives diagnosis
  in 85% of jundiced patients.

Indications:

    dilatation of bile ducts not seen on
    cholangiography in suspected gallstones

    to decide whether persistent symptoms
    after biliary tract surgery are due to stricture
    or overlooked stones

    to distinguish gallbladder disease from
    pancreatic or gastroduodenal disease

allows removal of gallstones through sphincterotomy

may show small stones in recurrent acute pancreatitis

ultrasound

indications

- to detect gallstones in non-functioning gallbladder on cholecystography
- to pick up very small stones – down to 3 mm diameter
- differential diagnosis of jaundice
- good demonstration of intrahepatic ducts
- preferable to radiology in pregnant women and in children

radio-isotope imaging (technetium Tc 99 m)

- can be used in jaundiced patients
- can pick up acute cholecystitis – no opacification of gallbladder within 1 hour

CT scan

not very helpful so far in picking up gallstones – nuclear magnetic resonance (NMR) may be better

liver function tests

- alkaline phosphatase more sensitive than serum bilirubin in indicating obstruction of CBD
- serum bilirubin and alkaline phosphatase higher in obstruction of CBD than in obstruction of cystic duct

differential diagnosis of biliary colic/cholecystitis

acute pancreatitis
- patient usually very ill with evidence of circulatory collapse and shock
- epigastric pain radiating through to back
- vomiting profuse
- may be past history of alcoholism
- tests

  serum amylase ↑ most important – > 1875 iu/litre is diagnostic

  serum Ca ↓ – bad prognosis

  blood sugar ↑

perforated peptic ulcer
- past history of indigestion related to food (80%)
- upper abdominal board-like rigidity
- pelvic tenderness on rectal examination
- development of ileus → silent abdominal distension
- tests – plain X-ray abdomen in erect position → air under diaphragm (seen in 70% of cases of perforation)

acute appendicitis (especially retrocaecal)
- no history of flatulent dyspepsia
- pain initially epigastric → right iliac fossa
- retrocaecal appendix → pain in right loin
- tenderness, guarding, rigidity in right iliac fossa
- rebound tenderness may be present
- right hip flexed with retrocaecal appendix
- tests

  X-ray abdomen may show

  soft tissue shadow RIF

  fluid level in caecum

  blurred psoas shadow

  laparotomy often required to decide

right renal colic due to stone
- pain typically in right loin radiating to right groin
- associated urinary symptoms

    frequency

    dysuria

    haematuria
- tenderness over kidney in loin with tenderness and rigidity along line of ureter
- tests

    urine – may show blood

    plain X-ray – radio-opaque stone (80% cases)

    i.v.p. – confirms intrarenal opacity

    cystoscopy – no urine from blocked ureter

perforated colonic carcinoma (hepatic flexure)
- no history of flatulent dyspepsia
- recent alteration of bowels
- passage of blood p.r.
- history of loss of weight
- mass may be felt in right upper quadrant
- tests

    plain X-ray for

    gas under diaphragm

    fluid levels due to intestinal obstruction

    laparotomy probably necessary

myocardial infarction
- may cause acute epigastric pain
- may be previous history of angina
- pain may radiate up to throat and down arms
- cardiac arrhythmias may be present
- abdominal examination

    no tenderness or Murphy's sign

    no rigidity
- tests – e.c.g.

acute porphyria

- rare condition
- may be precipitated by drugs
    - barbiturates
    - tranquillizers
    - oral hypoglycaemics
- constipation prominent feature
- other features
    - polyneuritis
    - mental disturbances
    - skin photosensitivity
- tests
    - let fresh urine stand → dark red
    - porphobilinogen found in urine

MANAGEMENT

issues

- silent gallstones – what to do?
- who needs cholecystectomy?
- who needs 'oral dissolution'?
- how to manage symptoms?
- how to manage complications?

'silent' gallstones

- only 'silent' until detected
- if left
    - 50% will have cholecystectomy within 20 years
    - 25% will develop serious complications
- most surgeons recommend elective prophylactic cholecystectomy provided patients are young and otherwise fit
- elderly patients should be treated conservatively
- medical dissolution treatment can be tried only with cholesterol stones

- remove gallbladder if gallstones and/or acute cholecystitis discovered accidentally during laparotomy for some other reason
- nevertheless 'silent' gallstones are found at autopsy of about one in four to five of adults without being detected in life

symptomatic gallstones

- biliary colic → elective cholecystectomy
- acute cholecystitis
    - conservative treatment first – analgesics, i.v. fluids
    - early elective cholecystectomy
- acute suppurative cholangitis
    - symptoms
        - high fever
        - progressive jaundice
        - increasing local signs over gallbladder
    - treatment
        - adequate hydration
        - antibiotics
        - urgent drainage of common bile duct
        - fatal without surgery
- empyema of gallbladder, perforation or peritonitis – urgent operation after adequate preceeding resuscitation measures
- biliary – enteric fistulae – elective repair operation

cholecystectomy

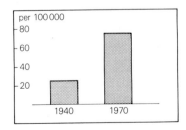

- increasing rates ×3 (per 100 000) in Bristol from 1940 to 1970[28]
- highest rates of increase in males and in young (under 30)

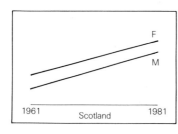

- in *Scotland*, 1961–1981, cholecystectomy rates increased[24]

    females × 2

    males × 3

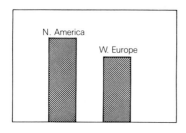

- cholecystectomy rates vary nationally – higher in *N. America* than in *W. Europe*[30]
- mortality of operation < 1%

postcholecystectomy problems

- stones may be left in common bile duct and may lead to

    recurrent biliary colic

    jaundice

    cholangitis

    pancreatitis

- always do operative cholangiogram to check for stones in CBD and if so they must be removed
- stones found postoperatively in CBD by cholangiography can be treated by

    T tube washout with saline

    removal with a special catheter through the T tube

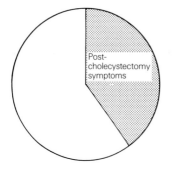

- 40% may still have symptoms after cholecystectomy

    if biliary colic, repeat radiology

    if vague abdominal symptoms, treat with antacids and reassurance

- there may be an increased risk of *cancer of the colon* after cholecystectomy

166

medical dissolution therapy

- indications
    - silent gallstones
    - infrequent symptoms
    - operation contraindicated
    - patient declines operation
- contraindications
    - radio-opaque gallstones
    - non-functioning gallbladder
    - very obese patients – excessive cholesterol secretion into bile
- two preparations
    - chenodeoxycholic acid (CDCA) (Chendol)
    - ursodeoxycholic acid (UDCA) (Destolit) less likely to cause diarrhoea than CDCA
- acts by reducing the cholesterol concentration in the bile relative to bile acids and phospholipids
- slow-acting – may take up to 5 years
- only 13.5% stones dissolve within 2 years
- dose
    - CDCA : 15 mg/kg single dose at bedtime
    - UDCA : 10 mg/kg single dose at bedtime
    - continue at least 2 years
    - continue until 3 months after stone is dissolved
- side-effects
    - diarrhoea – more with CDCA
    - pruritis
    - minor transient hepatic abnormalities
- additional treatment
    - low cholesterol diet
    - high fibre diet
- recurrence of gallstones after successful dissolution up to 70% 5 years after treatment – may mean long term maintenance treatment required

Useful practical points

- the presence of flatulent dyspepsia is as frequent in those without chronic gallbladder disease and gallstones as it is in those with the condition, so is of no diagnostic help

- since both peptic ulcer and chronic gallbladder disease are common conditions and often coexist, demonstration of the one condition should not lead to forgetting to check for the other in patients with an acute onset of upper abdominal pain

- biliary 'colic' is a misnomer – the pain is almost always constant and not 'colicky'

- the urine should always be checked for the presence of bile pigments in any patient with acute upper abdominal pain

- herpes zoster is rarely considered as a cause of unexplained pain in the right upper quadrant since the pain may antedate the typical vesicular rash by several days

- medical dissolution therapy for gallstones is not 'an easy way out' – it is a long, arduous and often ineffective treatment

10

IRRITABLE BOWEL
SYNDROME (IBS)

WHAT IS IT?

- IBS is a 'new-old' condition – under different labels it has been described for over a century
- it is the commonest gastrointestinal disorder in the Western world
- previously known as

   membranous enteritis (1871)

   mucous colitis (1906)

   neurogenic mucous colitis (1928)

   spastic colon (1928)

   nervous diarrhoea (1940)

symptoms

not a distinct pathological entity but is a collection of *symptoms*. Cardinal symptoms

- abdominal pain
- alteration of bowel habit

pain

- cramplike, colicky, nagging aching or burning
- most often epigastric or LIF – can be anywhere else in abdomen (Figure 10.1)
- site of pain frequently varies in same patient
- may be relieved by passing flatus or defaecation
- may be worse after eating or alcohol
- may be periodic, lasting for a few weeks or a few months at a time

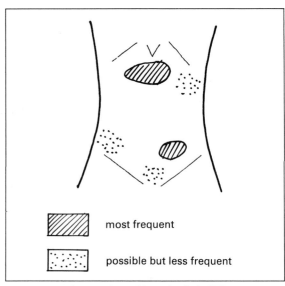

Figure 10.1   *Sites of pain in IBS*

	▨ most frequent
	⁛ possible but less frequent

bowels

- loose stools (diarrhoea)
- constipation
- may alternate diarrhoea/constipation
- may be painless diarrhoea (10%)

faeces

- pellet-like ('rabbit' or 'goat' 'droppings')
- ribbon or pencil-like
- may contain excessive mucus
- may be watery as in painless diarrhoea
- never contains blood unless associated piles

other abdominal symptoms

- abdominal distension
- rumbling (borborygmi)
- postprandial fullness
- belching
- heartburn
- nausea

clinical examination	• a thorough examination is necessary in every case
	to exclude organic disease
	to reassure the patient
	• possible findings are shown in Figure 10.2
	• sigmoidoscopy essential
	to exclude organic disease
	may show slight hyperaemia in IBS
	may show excessive mucus in IBS
	may sometimes show contraction rings
	air insufflation may cause excessive pain

clinical examination

- a thorough examination is necessary in every case

    to exclude organic disease

    to reassure the patient
- possible findings are shown in Figure 10.2
- sigmoidoscopy essential

    to exclude organic disease

    may show slight hyperaemia in IBS

    may show excessive mucus in IBS

    may sometimes show contraction rings

    air insufflation may cause excessive pain

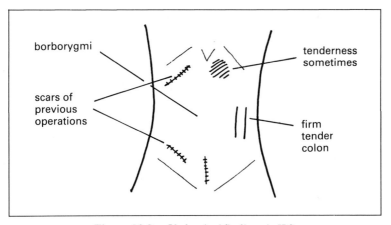

Figure 10.2   *Abdominal findings in IBS*

WHO GETS IT WHEN?

- a condition of developed Western societies, possibly due to fibre-depleted diets
- may be associated with 'diathesis' of sensitive, tense, anxious personality
- F > M

age – onset

- in young adults[31]

age – prevalence	• peak of symptoms 20–50
	• occurs throughout adult life
	• possible relationship to 'little bellyachers'

suggested that children with recurrent abdominal pains, 'little bellyachers', may become 'big bellyachers' with adult IBS

| frequency | • suggested that up to 20% of adults have features of IBS[32] |

| *district general hospital* | • up to one third of all OP gastroenterological referrals are for IBS |

| *general practice* | practice population of 2500 (UK): IBS – annual numbers |

new cases (incidence)	5–7
patients consulting (prevalence)	25–30

WHAT HAPPENS?

- there should be *no mortality* from IBS
- *morbidity*

  symptoms (abdominal pain/discomfort and bowel changes) may be persistent and continuous or intermittent

  peak of symptoms is at 20–60 years

  one third of patients become symptom-free for variable periods of weeks to years

  up to one half of IBS sufferers eventually *cease to suffer symptoms* after 10–15 years of activity

  only 5% eventually develop intractable symptoms

  some IBS symptoms merge into '*diverticular disease*' with age

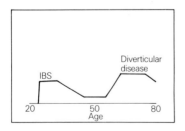

WHAT TO DO?

issues
- uncertain disorder of uncertain cause, uncertain course and outcome
- possible aetiological factors

    dietary – lack of roughage (fibre)

    post-infective, e.g. dysentery

    hormonal – disturbance of gut hormones

    disturbance of autonomic nervous system

    lactose intolerance – small number

    psychogenic factors   stress

                    depression

                    personality change
- with such a common vague syndrome it is easy and dangerous to use 'IBS' label for any ill-defined GI symptoms and miss dangerous treatable diseases such as cancer

diagnosis
- by careful *history and examination* with positive and negative features
- by exclusory *investigations*

    faeces

        occult blood

        parasites

        if stool weight > 300 g/day organic disease is likely to be present

    sigmoidoscopy

    rectal biopsy to exclude occult inflammation

    colonoscopy

    barium enema

    small bowel enema especially to exclude Crohn's disease

    an ESR is useful to exclude neoplastic disease
- IBS has to be a diagnosis of exclusion with positive symptoms and minimal or no signs

- features which should raise suspicion of organic disease rather than IBS are:

  significant weight loss

  elderly patient developing symptoms for the first time

  unexpected physical signs, e.g. abdominal mass

  blood in the stools – frank or occult

  fever

  anaemia

  raised ESR

differential diagnosis

diverticular disease

- pain confined to LIF in 90% of cases
- rectal bleeding may occur
- may flare up → diverticulitis

  fever

  increased pain in LIF

  tender mass in LIF

  rectal tenderness

  may develop   abscess

                        perforation

                        peritonitis

                        obstruction

                        fistula

                            bladder

                            vagina

- tests

  sigmoidoscopy

  barium enema

ulcerative colitis

- younger patients (20–40)
- bloody diarrhoea

- constitutional symptoms
    fever
    weight loss
    malaise
- systemic signs
    eyes
    joints/spine
    skin
    liver
- tests
    proctosigmoidoscopy and biopsy
    barium enema

Crohn's disease

- like ulcerative colitis but less rectal bleeding
- perianal signs
    blue induration
    abscesses
    fistulae
- mass in RIF common
- tests
    as for ulcerative colitis but often difficulty in distinguishing between these two conditions

carcinoma colon

- *recent* change in bowel habits in middle-aged or elderly
    constipation
    diarrhoea
- rectal bleeding
- weight loss common
- symptoms of anaemia common
- may develop obstruction
- mass may be felt in abdomen

- tests

  sigmoidoscopy

  barium enema

  colonoscopy for proximal cancer

chronic mesenteric ischaemia
- recurrent postprandial colicky *periumbilical* pain
- usually 15–30 min after eating
- diarrhoea associated with pain
- signs of arteriosclerosis elsewhere
- tests

  barium meal/follow through – may show 'thumbprinting'

  superior mesenteric artery angiography is definitive test

TREATMENT

explanation
- explanation to patient

  nature of the pain

  stress benign nature and *not* cancer

  doesn't need an operation

  there are no complications

  avoid stress if possible

  state measures to help symptoms

  avoid purgatives

  always sympathy and reassurance

investigation of GI tract
- it is necessary to have a thorough investigation of the gastrointestinal tract only once – repeated investigations, especially at different hospitals, can only exacerbate symptoms and increase anxiety

diet	• avoid any food or drink known to exacerbate symptoms
	• increased roughage useful where repeated colic occurs due to colonic spasm
	leafy vegetables
	fruit
	wholemeal bread
	• a low milk (lactose) diet can be tried in difficult cases in view of possible intolerance of milk products
bulking agents	• useful if severe constipation
	• products available
	Isogel 10 ml once/twice daily after meals
	Normacol 5–10 ml once/twice daily after meals
	Cologel 5–15 ml t.d.s. after meals
	• maintain adequate fluid intake to avoid intestinal obstruction
bran products	• natural product – in wholemeal bread, high bran cereal and raw bran
	• useful if severe constipation
	• may be unpalatable
	• may cause excessive wind
antispasmodics	• anticholinergic drugs (Pro-Banthine, Buscopan) should not be used because the high dose required leads to side-effects.
	dry mouth
	retention of urine
	blurring of vision
	• mebeverine (Colofac) has a direct relaxant effect on spastic intestinal muscle and is well worth trying – dose 135–270 mg (1–2 tabs) q.d.s.

                                       • peppermint oil (Colpermin) sometimes helps.

psychotropic drugs   • anxiolytic and antidepressive drugs should
                                         only be used when anxiety and depression are
                                         major factors
                                       • combination of *Motival* (once daily), *Colofac*
                                         (540 mg daily) and *Fybogel* (ispaghula 7 g
                                         daily) may be effective in IBS[33]

antidiarrhoeal drugs   • useful if diarrhoea is predominant – especially
                                         in the 'painless diarrhoea' type of IBS
                                       • codeine phosphate 30–60 mg t.d.s. is effective,
                                         but long term use can lead to dependence
                                       • Imodium 4–8 mg daily
                                       • Lomotil 5 mg 6-hourly
                                       • side-effects
                                             dizziness
                                             sedation (codeine)
                                             rashes
                                             intestinal ileus

other treatment   • hypnotherapy
                                       • psychotherapy
                                       • behavioural therapy
                                       • little evidence of benefit

---

Summary of treatment of IBS

- explanation and reassurance
- avoid obvious food/drink precipitants
- bulking agents to help pain/constipation
- mebeverine (Colofac) to relieve pain
- antidiarrhoeal drugs for painless diarrhoea

> *Useful practical points*
> - common condition
> - symptom–complex
> - no distinctive signs
> - diagnosis by exclusion
> - condition of young and middle-aged adults
> - one half cease to suffer symptoms
> - wide choice of therapies – uncertain benefits

11 ULCERATIVE COLITIS

WHAT IS IT?

- an inflammatory condition of the large bowel
- ranges from mild limited proctitis to severe extensive involvement of whole of colon
- main clinical features

    diarrhoea

    bleeding from the bowel

    general systemic illness

    extra-intestinal manifestations

causes unknown

causes unknown – possible factors:

- *transmissable infection* – unlikely

    bacterial

    virus

- *nutritional* – unlikely

    food allergy, e.g. milk

    toxic factor in food

- *psychosomatic* – difficult to evaluate whether the emotional disorder in patients is primary or secondary to the disease
- *immunological disturbance* – quite likely
- *heredity* – probably relevant (10%)

    HLA-B27 in 50–90% of patients with colitis or Crohn's when there is associated ankylosing spondylitis (control population 6–9%)

- *impairment of blood supply* – no good evidence

WHO GETS IT WHEN?

geographical distribution

- *more* prevalent: USA, Canada, Scandinavia, UK, W. Germany
- *less* prevalent: Africa, Asia, S. America, S. Europe[27]

genetic

- whites > blacks
- Jews > non-Jews
- Israeli-born Western Jews > North African and Asian Jews[34]

class, location, sex

- no social class differences
- no urban–rural differences
- sex distribution: F > M (marginally) 1:1.2

age – onset (incidence)

- can occur at any age but most often age 20–50

age – prevalence (cases)

- from age 20 onwards

family history

- increased likelihood of FH of ulcerative colitis and Crohn's disease

     applies to parents and siblings

     no increased likelihood in husband–wife
- increased incidence of ankylosing spondylitis in relatives
- onset of disease from affected families occurs at a younger age

frequency

- new cases (annual incidence): five per 100 000
- prevalence (cases in population): 100 per 100 000

general practice	practice population of 2500 (UK): annual numbers	
	New cases (incidence)	1 every 5 years
	Patients consulting (prevalence)	2–3

district general hospital	DGH with 250 000 persons: annual numbers	
	Admissions	25
	Patients under care	150

trends

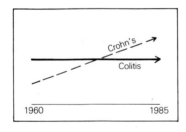

- no apparent increase in incidence of ulcerative colitis over past 25 years, but there has been an increase in Crohn's disease in developed countries

WHAT HAPPENS?

onset

- *gradual – mild*
  loose stools
  blood + mucus in the stools
  abdominal pain   lower abdomen or LIF
                           usually ache – colic less
                           relieved by defaecation
  tenesmus often due to proctitis
  general condition good
  anaemia from chronic blood loss

- *acute – severe*
  - diarrhoea + +
  - mucopus, blood in stools
  - poor general condition
    - anorexia
    - nausea and vomiting
    - weight loss +
    - profound weakness
    - tachycardia
    - fever
    - sweating
    - dehydration   dry skin and tongue
                             low eyeball tension
                             low blood pressure
    - electrolyte disturbance   K loss $\rightarrow$ arrhythmias
                                       Na loss $\rightarrow$ cramps, low BP
  - anaemic
- *toxic megacolon*
  - gravely ill
  - high swinging temperature
  - generalized abdominal pain
  - abdominal distension
  - rebound tenderness (peritonitis)
  - straight X-ray abdomen $\rightarrow$ colonic distension + +
  - high mortality

course
- *episodic – recurrent* (75% of cases)
  intermittent attacks over years
- *continuous – unremitting* (20%)
- *single attack* (5%)

complications and associated disorders

local (Figure 11.1)

- perforation → peritonitis
- haemorrhage
- ischiorectal abscess
- toxic megacolon
- cancer (20% after 20 years) (usually in ascending and transverse colon)

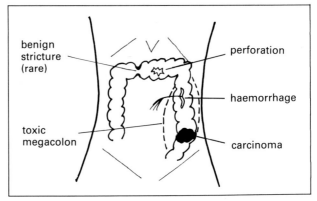

Figure 11.1   *Local complications of ulcerative colitis*

remote (Figure 11.2)

- *eyes* (5%)   episcleritis

          uveitis
- *mouth* (10%)   ulcers
- *skin* (5%)   erythema nodosum

          gangrenous pyoderma
- *joints* (25%)   polyarthritis

          ankylosing spondylitis

          sacroiliitis
- *liver* (2%)   cirrhosis

          cholangitis

          abnormal liver function tests (90%)
- *kidney* (less than 1%) – stones (especially after ileostomy)

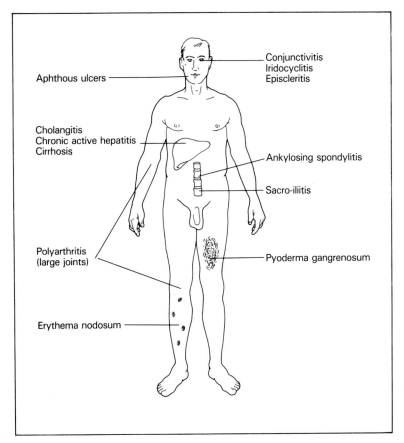

Figure 11.2 *Extra-intestinal complications of ulcerative colitis*

mortality

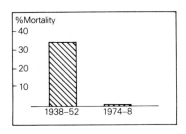

- *case fatality of severe attacks* from 34% (1938–52) to less than 1% (1974–8: Oxford)[34]
- ulcerative colitis diminishes *life expectancy*

WHAT TO DO?

issues

- initial presentation may be vague and difficult to diagnose
- accurate diagnosis important
- long term care usually required (lifelong)
- complications frequent
- appreciable morbidity and mortality

differential diagnosis

Crohn's disease

- this is the major differential diagnosis

Clinical feature	Colitis	Crohn's disease
Pain	lower abdomen	central abdomen
	LIF	RIF
Diarrhoea	severe	moderate
Belching	frequent	infrequent
Abdominal mass	no	frequent – RIF
		central
Perianal disease	rare	frequent
Fistulae	rare	frequent
Malabsorption	no	frequent
Mouth ulcers	rare	frequent

carcinoma rectum

- older patients
- progressive symptoms
- constipation rather than diarrhoea
- abdominal or rectal mass

dysentery

- *bacillary* (Shigella – shiga, flexneri, sonnei)

    more likely in institutions

    may be mild or very acute

    stools small with a lot of pus

    arthritis or iritis may occur

    diagnose by faecal culture

- *amoebic* (Entamoeba histolytica)
  - usually chronic
  - pain may resemble D.U.
  - often constipation alternating with diarrhoea
  - stools very offensive
  - tender mainly in RIF
  - may affect liver – enlarged and tender
  - examine fresh stool for amoebae

ischaemic colitis

- postprandial colicky central abdominal pain (20–30 min p.c.)
- diarrhoea with the pain
- signs of arteriosclerosis
  - radial thickening
  - brachial tortuosity
  - absent foot pulses
  - abdominal aortic murmur
  - carotid murmur
- X-ray abdomen may show 'thumbprinting'
- diagnose by mesenteric angiography

pseudomembranous colitis

- recent antibiotic especially ampicillin and clindamycin
- 7–11 days after treatment
- bloody watery stools
- examine stools for *Clostridium difficile* and its toxins
- sigmoidoscopy may show membrane

piles

- constipation frequent
- bleeding at end of defaecation and not intimately mixed with stool
- anal pain and irritation frequent
- piles may prolapse
- proctoscopy/sigmoidoscopy helpful

investigations

stool examination
- exclude pathogens
  shigellae

  amoebae

  campylobacter
- *C. difficile* toxin

blood
- blood count polymorph leukocytosis

  anaemia
- ESR high
- electrolytes low sodium

  low potassium
- liver function abnormal if hepatic involvement

proctosigmoidoscopy
- mild – hyperaemia, oedema
- moderate – red granular mucosa – contact bleeding
- severe – ulcerated mucosa – spontaneous bleeding

colonoscopy
- no place in routine diagnosis
- helpful in distinguishing Crohn's disease
- assesses extent of disease prior to surgery
- to detect carcinoma in longstanding colitis

rectal biopsy
- mucosa affected
- plasma cells, polymorphs, eosinophils
- mucus depletion, gland destruction
- crypt abscesses

X-rays	• plain – may show ragged, ulcerated mucosa in dilated segment of bowel
	• barium enema
	shows extent of disease
	mucosal ulceration seen
	shortening and narrowing colon
	'collarstud' ulcers
	pseudopolyps

TREATMENT

acute severe attack (hospital admission)

- replace plasma volume – saline, plasma
- blood transfusion if severe anaemia
- parenteral nutrition
- prednisolone 60–80 mg/day
- hydrocortisone enemas 100 mg b.d.
- possibly erythromycin

mild attack (home treatment)

- sulphasalazine
    1 g q.d.s. initially
    0.5 g q.d.s. for maintenance
- steroid p.r.
    hydrocortisone
        suppository
        colifoam
        enema
    prednisolone
        suppository
        enema

long-term maintenance treatment

- *sulphasalazine* 0.5 g q.d.s.

  suitable for most patients to prevent relapses

  side-effects   headache

  gastrointestinal upset

  rashes

  arthralgia

  blood

     haemolysis

     leukopenia

     agranulocytosis

- *oral steroids*

  after acute severe attack continue oral steroids 4–6 weeks in reducing dose

  long term steroids are rarely necessary and potentially hazardous

  side-effects   weight gain

  fluid retention

     oedema

     hypertension

  diabetes

  hypokalaemia

  acute gastritis

  osteoporosis, especially spine

  mental disturbance ·(psychosis)

- *azathioprine*

  not effective in acute exacerbation

  may help to prevent relapses

  may produce bone marrow depression with pancytopenia

- *sodium cromoglycate* (Nalcrom)

  may be useful in reducing relapses if the patient can't take sulphasalazine

other general aspects of treatment

- *diet* – well-balanced

  adequate calories/proteins/vitamins/ minerals

  reduce fibre content (less fruit and vegetables)

  occasional milk intolerance
- *anaemia* – usually chronic iron deficiency due to blood loss – treat with iron
- *antidiarrhoeal drugs*

  codeine phosphate 30–60 mg t.d.s

  Lomotil 5 mg 6-hourly

  Imodium 2 mg up to 8/day
- *good doctor/patient rapport*

  simple clear explanation

  realistic expectations from treatment

  sympathy

  encouragement

indications for surgery

- local complications

  perforation

  haemorrhage

  toxic megacolon

  benign stricture
- severe unresponsive acute attack after 5 days treatment
- chronic unresponsive symptomatic disease
- neoplasia

  precarcinomatous change on colonoscopy

  longstanding pancolitis (> 10 y)

  developed carcinoma

prognosis

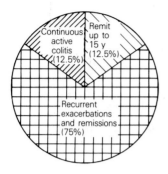

Continuous active colitis (12.5%)

Remit up to 15 y (12.5%)

Recurrent exacerbations and remissions (75%)

- adverse factors

    elderly patient (> 60 y)

    very young onset

    severe initial attack – 50% die within the next 20 years

    extensive colonic involvement

- risk of carcinoma

    particularly with pancolitis 10% at 10 years

    rises by 10% per 10 years thereafter

- mortality of severe acute attacks should be less than 5% in the best centres

- 5-year mortality 5–15%

- causes of death

    acute   massive haemorrhage

              toxic megacolon

              systemic infection

              pulmonary embolism

    late   cancer of colon

Useful practical points

- ulcerative colitis is an uncommon condition of young adults which has a significant morbidity and mortality
- there is an increasing risk of carcinoma of the colon if the whole of the colon is affected for at least 10 years
- it is difficult to differentiate between ulcerative colitis and Crohn's disease – the most helpful clinical points in Crohn's disease are infrequent rectal bleeding, a mass in the RIF and perianal disease
- if ulcerative colitis seems to follow an atypical course always think of Crohn's disease
- don't forget to enquire for the systemic complications of ulcerative colitis affecting eyes, joints, spine, skin and liver
- mild ulcerative colitis can be treated at home by the general practitioner with local steroid enemas and sulphasalazine; a severe attack requires urgent hospital treatment with intravenous fluids, including blood transfusions, and intravenous steroids
- the prognosis of surgically-treated ulcerative colitis (for local complications or intractability to medical treatment) is good – that for Crohn's disease is bad
- ulcerative colitis requires lifelong care and supervision

12　DIVERTICULAR DISEASE

WHAT IS IT?

- mucosal herniations of colon accompanied by hypertrophy of muscles. Most in sigmoid and descending colon (95%)

- a well-nigh 'normal' (inevitable) condition associated with ageing

- majority never have symptoms from their diverticulae

- *symptoms* when present are those of bowel dysfunction and complications, as perforation-infection, bleeding and obstruction

- *causes* uncertain, but popular current theory is that it is a consequence of deficiency in diet of bran and other bulk roughage

- persons with colonic diverticulae have higher than expected *disease associations* (Figure 12.1)

    appendicitis

    large bowel cancer

    haemorrhoids

    gallbladder disease

    hiatus hernia

    peptic ulcers

---

complications

perforation

peritonitis

bleeding

obstruction

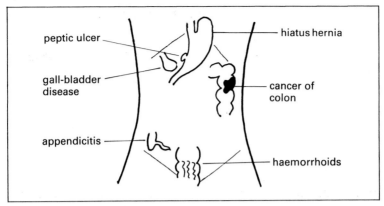

Figure 12.1   *Associations of diverticular disease*

WHO GETS IT WHEN?[34, 35]

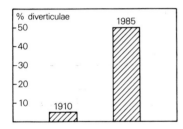

- difficult to be certain what proportion of population has colonic diverticulae – data come from autopsies and barium enema examinations

- autopsy   5% in 1910

        50% today

- rising trends of prevalence and mortality may be apparent rather than real and results of greater interest in and awareness of the condition

mortality rates

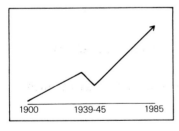

- mortality rates (by death certification) have increased steadily this century, with transient fall during World War II period (1939–1945)

age/sex

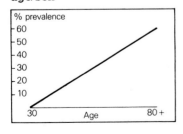

- *age prevalence* at autopsy shows progressive increase of diverticulae

    nil at 30 years old

    60% over 80 years old

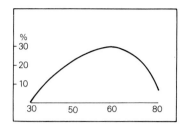

- *age at onset of symptoms*
  maximal at 50–70 years
  (but majority do *not* have symptoms)
- probably M = F

geographical distribution

- 40% more frequent in Western societies than in developing countries, e.g. Africa
- *incidence* increases in Africans or Japanese if they settle in the West – probably due to reduction of dietary fibre

Trends		
+ +	+	−
Western developed countries	increasing	*Developing countries*
USA W. Europe Australia	Japan	Africa India Far East

Data: ref 27

distribution of diverticulae

- sigmoid and descending colon – 95% of cases in Western society
- caecum and ascending colon – Eastern races (Japan; Hawaii)
- other rarer sites
  oesophagus
  stomach
  duodenum
  small bowel

frequency

rates shown here are of those presenting symptoms

general practice

practice population of 2500 (UK)

Patients consulting (prevalence) per year	10

district general hospital (estimated)

DGH with 250 000 population	
Annual admissions	50
Attending OPD	250

- increases in admissions and OP referrals over the past 25 years probably because of longer living population, more awareness and more investigations.

WHAT HAPPENS?

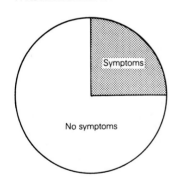

- it is likely that the majority of persons with diverticulae *do not ever have symptoms* – perhaps up to 75%
- *symptoms*

    may occur in the absence of acute inflammation – *painful diverticular disease.*

    may be due to acute inflammation – *diverticulitis*

    may be due to *complications*

painful diverticular disease

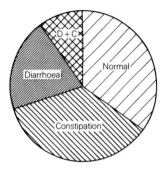

- abdominal pain
    colicky
    usually left-sided
    lasts 1–3 days
    settles with rest
- alteration of bowel habit
    intermittent diarrhoea   (20%)
    diarrhoea/constipation   (10%)
    constipation   (35%)
    normal   (35%)
- symptoms resembling irritable bowel syndrome
    abdominal distension
    flatulence
    rumbling
    heartburn

acute diverticulitis (Figure 12.2)

- less than 10% of patients with diverticulae
- sudden onset lower abdominal pain ('acute abdomen')
- tenderness and guarding LIF
- inflammatory mass may be in LIF

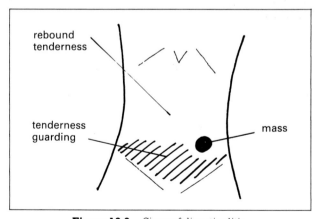

Figure 12.2   *Signs of diverticulitis*

DIVERTICULAR DISEASE

- high fever
- constipation
- tests

  polymorph leukocytosis

  high E S R
- differentiate from painful (non-inflammatory) diverticular disease by raised white cell count and high E S R.

complications (Figure 12.3)

- types[35]
- perforation, abscess, peritonitis (25% of complications)

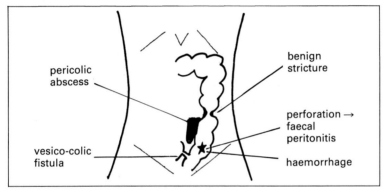

Figure 12.3   *Complications of acute diverticulitis*

  fistula (5%)

  bladder → pneumaturia

  vagina

  small bowel

  renal tract

  bleeding   (25%)

  obstruction   (5%)

  other e.g. portal; pyaemial   (5%)

- hospital admission essential
- commonest cause of severe colonic haemorrhage in elderly
- 40% mortality with perforation leading to faecal peritonitis

natural history (hospital admissions)

no further symptoms	45%
mild symptoms	22%
severe symptoms	3%
death from diverticular disease	5%
death from other causes	20%

Data: ref. 35 (5–25-year follow-up)

WHAT TO DO?

issues

- finding large bowel diverticulae in elderly persons does not denote a 'disease'
- most are, and will always be, asymptomatic
- 'diverticular disease' becomes a problem when it produces symptoms and/or complications
- if it is believed that diverticulae are 'caused' by dietary deficiencies of bran etc, then national diets must be changed to prevent them
- active treatment of diverticulae is necessary for complications
- it is important not to turn a normal anatomical condition of ageing into a universal disease

differential diagnosis

beware of over-easy labelling as 'diverticular disease'

carcinoma of the colon

- progressive symptoms
- shorter history
- progressive weight loss
- palpable abdominal or rectal mass (painless)

- tests

    sigmoidoscopy + biopsy

    colonoscopy

    barium enema

    laparotomy

  N.B. cancer of colon may coexist with diverticulosis

ulcerative colitis

- younger age group
- bloody diarrhoea prominent
- pain usually slight
- tests

    sigmoidoscopy + biopsy

    barium enema

Crohn's disease

- younger age group
- right-sided abdominal pain
- mass in RIF
- perianal disease frequent
- ankylosing spondylitis (20%)
- tests

    colonoscopy + biopsy

    small bowel enema

tubo-ovarian disease

- pain lower abdomen + lower back
- worse before periods
- vaginal discharge
- dyspareunia
- cervix and tubes tender p.v.

chronic urinary infection

- pain in loins as well as left side abdomen
- urinary symptoms
  - frequency
  - dysuria
- suprapubic tenderness
- haematuria may be present
- tests
  - urine examination
  - i.v.p.
  - cystoscopy and retrograde pyelogram

investigations

indications

- to confirm diverticulosis (Figure 12.4)
- to exclude carcinoma of colon (may coexist with diverticulosis)

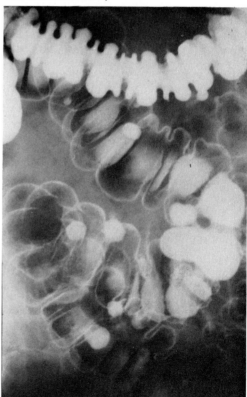

Figure 12.4 *Barium enema showing multiple diverticulae*

DIVERTICULAR DISEASE

tests

- sigmoidoscopy – to exclude cancer rectum or rectosigmoid
- colonoscopy – to exclude more proximal cancer of the colon
- barium enema

  characteristic diverticulae

  narrowing and rigidity

  loss of haustration

  may show fistulae   bladder

                                     vagina

                                     small bowel

                                     ureter

TREATMENT

- *diet*

  high fibre diet   fruit

                            vegetables

                            100% wholemeal bread

  avoid refined flour and sugar
- *bran supplements*   miller's bran

                                   All-bran cereal

                                   Shredded Wheat

                                   muesli

                                   bran tablets (for holiday use)
- *bulking agents*   methylcellulose (Celevac, Cologel)

                               ispaghula husk (Fybogel, Isogel)

                               sterculia (Normacol)

(*N.B.* A high fibre bran diet relieves 90% of the symptoms of uncomplicated diverticular disease)

COMPLICATIONS

acute diverticulitis
- gastric suction
- i.v. fluids
- antibiotics (metronidazole, ampicillin)
- pethidine (*not* morphine – increases spasm)
- if fails to subside → proximal colostomy followed by later resection

pericolic abscess
- initial drainage and proximal colostomy
- later resection diseased bowel segment and close colostomy

perforation
- emergency resection
  terminal colostomy
  closure of rectal stump

        or
- temporary proximal colostomy
  exteriorize diseased colon
  later resection

fistulae
- partial colonic resection and repair of fistulous opening
- staged operation best

stricture
- bowel resection

sigmoid myotomy
- in local muscular hypertrophy
- longitudinal division of circular muscle
- relieves pain due to bowel spasm

(*N.B. Exploratory laparotomy always required if the diagnosis of carcinoma of colon cannot be satisfactorily excluded any other way*)

PROGNOSIS
- good in great majority
- problems are caused by complications

Useful practical points

- very common
- part of normal ageing
- may result from insufficient bulk in Western diets
- most are asymptomatic
- symptoms from dysfunction of large bowel may be from diet or from the diverticular disorder
- major problems arise from intra-abdominal complications
- beware of coincidental cancer
- management depends on views of causes
  - ? nil
  - ? diet (bran +)
  - ? other
  - ? surgery
- good prognosis

13   DIABETES

- condition of permanently disordered carbohydrate metabolism with a relative or absolute deficiency of insulin
- cardinal symptoms

    thirst

    polyuria

    loss of weight
- diagnosis by blood sugar level (WHO criteria)

    fasting > 8 mmol/l

    2 h after glucose load (75 g in adults, 1.75 g/ kg children) > 11 mmol/l

    random in symptomatic patient > 11 mmol/l
- no single cause, probably multifactorial

    genetic – predisposition HLA, DR3, DR4, B8, B15

    immunological – insulin antibodies
                        sometimes

    environmental

    viral infection
- two clinical types

    Type I – insulin-dependent (IDDM)

        severe – often in juveniles

    Type II – non-insulin-dependent (NIDDM)

        mild – mature onset

- although diabetes can occur at any time it is a condition that increases with age
- M > F in juveniles
- F > M in mature onset (type II)
- *causes* – uncertain but may be a form of auto-immune disorder
- *family history* – one fifth of diabetics have a diabetic relative (more so in type II)
- *racial*

    more than expected in

    > Jews

    > Asians/Indians

    > West Indians

    > Malayans

    less than expected in
    Maltese
- *obesity* a factor in type II

frequency

- ½ million known diabetics in UK
- ½ million undiagnosed diabetics or potential diabetics in UK

general practice

general practice with 2500 population: annual numbers	
New diabetics: (incidence)	3
Known diabetics	25
(Undiagnosed diabetics	25)
Diabetics on	
insulin	10
drugs	10
diet	5

district general hospital

DGH 250 000 population: diabetics

Diabetics in district	2500
Attending hospital clinics (On insulin)	1500 (1000)

WHAT HAPPENS?

mortality

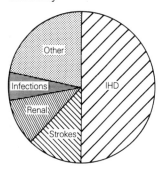

morbidity

- *life expectancy* is reduced by one third
- *causes of death*

  ischaemic heart disease

  50%   (27% in non-diabetics)

  strokes

  12%   (12% in non-diabetics)

  renal

  10%   (1% in non-diabetics)

  infections

  6%   (2% in non-diabetics)

  ketoacidosis

  1%

- *mortality trends: 1897–1961*

  over 60s (fall × 2)

  40–60 (fall × 11)

  20–40 (fall × 200)

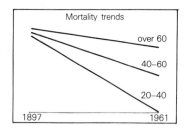

N.B. greatest benefits for young diabetics[36]

- most diabetics do *NOT* develop major serious complications
- *complications* when they do occur are directly related to duration of disease and age of diabetic: they are shown in Figure 13.1
- influence of *control* (good/bad) is difficult to assess but is thought to be relevant in the development of diabetic neuropathy, nephropathy and retinopathy (microvascular disease)

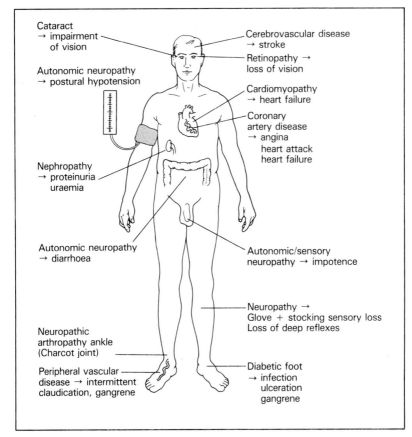

Figure 13.1 *Complications of diabetes*

eyes

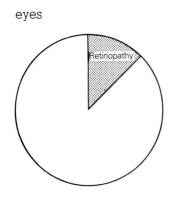

- diabetic retinopathy is commonest cause of blindness in 30–64-year-olds in the UK and accounts for 14% of all new blind registrations

- 8% of diabetics are *blind*

  F > M in mature onset (Type II)

  M > F in juvenile onset (Type I)

- half of those blind are *over 70*

- four fifths of those blind are *over 60*

- one fifth of those blind are *under 60*

- *retinopathy*

  10–15% of all diabetics

  the features are shown in Figure 13.2

  closely related to duration of diabetes – seldom seen < 5 y disease

  65% affected after 15–20 y of disease

  note: one third with 21-year+ diabetes do *not* have retinopathy

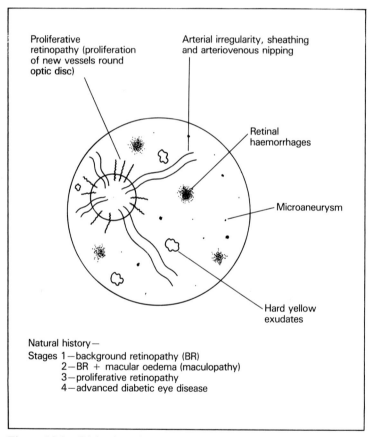

Proliferative retinopathy (proliferation of new vessels round optic disc)

Arterial irregularity, sheathing and arteriovenous nipping

Retinal haemorrhages

Microaneurysm

Hard yellow exudates

Natural history—

Stages 1—background retinopathy (BR)
      2—BR + macular oedema (maculopathy)
      3—proliferative retinopathy
      4—advanced diabetic eye disease

Figure 13.2 *Diabetic retinopathy – all stages*

kidneys

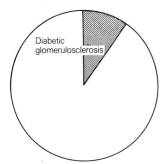

Diabetic
glomerulosclerosis

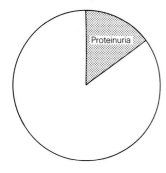

Proteinuria

diabetic arterial disease

*kidneys – diabetic glomerulosclerosis
(Kimmelstiel–Wilson)*

- more frequent in insulin-dependent
  (Type I)
- persistent proteinuria indicates
  nephropathy
- present in 10% attenders at a hospital
  diabetic clinic
- 10% of *deaths* in diabetics are from
  nephropathy
- directly related to

  age – prognosis worse in older patients

  sex – more common in men

  duration – 10 years +
- associated with retinopathy in virtually all
  patients with advanced glomerulosclerosis
- after 20 years of diabetes

  15% have *proteinuria*

  75% of these are in terminal renal failure
  after 10 years of continuous proteinuria

- *peripheral vascular disease*

  absent foot pulses – 8%

  intermittent claudication – 3%

  gangrene – less than 1%

  arterial calcification common in X-rays
- *ischaemic heart disease*

  50% diabetics *die* from ischaemic heart
  disease (twice the rate in non-diabetics);
  may be due to coexistence of small vessel
  disease in the heart and impaired
  myocardial cell metabolism

diabetic neuropathy

- types

    polyneuropathy

    sensory

    autonomic

    mononeuropathy

    cranial nerves (III, V)

    femoral (amyotrophy)

    radiculopathy

    other isolated peripheral nerves

- autonomic neuropathy – effects

    diarrhoea

    postural hypotension

    impotence

    gustatory sweating

    bladder disturbance

    cardiac denervation

- pressure palsies more common in diabetes

    carpal tunnel syndrome

    ulnar nerve compression

    foot-drop

MANAGEMENT: WHAT RESULTS OF TREATMENT?

aims of treatment

- relief of symptoms – fatigue, thirst, polyuria, loss of weight

- prevent/delay complications – may be possible in retinopathy, neuropathy, nephropathy

- prolong life

Note: achievement of absolute and constant normal blood sugar levels is rarely possible

considerations involved in management

- treatment of diabetes
- organization and implementation of long-term care and supervision
- responsibilities of

    diabetic self-care

    GP and primary health care team

    hospital specialties

types of treatment available

- diet (20%)
- oral drugs + diet (40%)
- insulin + diet (40%)

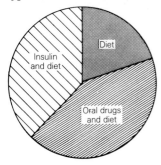

diet

- maintain habitual eating pattern if possible
- reduce total fat to about 30% of total calories
- reduce saturated fat (animal fat, dairy produce)
- low calorie diet for obese patients
- high fibre foods advisable

    wholemeal bread

    beans

    raw vegetables

    bran products

- children – review dietary needs with growth
- elderly – not too restrictive diet as it may precipitate dietary deficiencies

oral drugs

- indications

    hyperglycaemia and/or diabetic symptoms without ketonuria failing to respond to diet over 1 month

    elderly patients with mild diabetes

- drugs available

    Sulphonylureas

    tolbutamide (Rastinon) 250 mg – 1 g. b.d.

    chlorpropamide (Diabenese) 125–500 mg o.d.

    glibenclamide (Daonil, Euglycon) 2.5–15 mg o.d.

    Biguanides

    metformin (Glucophage) 500 mg t.d.s. – 850 mg b.d.

- side-effects

    gastrointestinal

    facial flushing after alcohol

    chlorpropamide mainly

    tolbutamide – less likely

    hypothyroidism (chlorpropamide)

    skin rashes

    paraesthesiae and weakness – rare

    lactic acidosis (metformin)

    reduced B_{12} absorption (metformin)

insulin

- indication – thirst, polyuria and ketonuria in non-obese patient
- types available

    short-acting: 6–8 h   Actrapid MC

                          Humilin S

    intermediate: 18–24 h   Monotard MC

                          Humilin I

long-acting: 30–36 h	Ultratard MC
mixtures: 2–24 h	Rapitard MC
	Mixtard 30/70

- single or multiple dose

  single dose

  elderly needing < 30 units/day

  patients rejecting multiple dose

  NIDDM failing with diet and tablets

  multiple dose

  best control for most patients

  twice daily most frequent regimen

  use mixture of short and intermediate action for each dose

- human or animal insulin – no evidence yet available that human insulin has any significant clinical advantages over highly purified (mono-component) beef or pork insulin

- pregnancy – always use highly-purified insulin since insulin antibodies from standard insulin can diffuse from the mother into the fetus and cause fetal pancreatic damage

- insulin lipoatrophy – treat by change to highly purified insulin

degrees of control of diabetes – all treatments

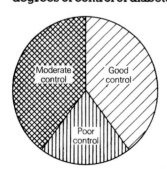

- good – blood sugar < 10 mmol/l – 40%
- moderate – blood sugar 10–19 mmol/l – 40%
- poor – blood sugar > 19 mmol/l – 20%

control with diet only

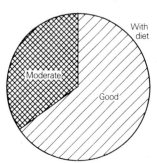

- good – 65%
- moderate – 35%

control with oral drugs + diet

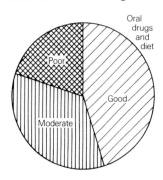

- good – 45%
- moderate – 35%
- poor – 20%

control with insulin + diet

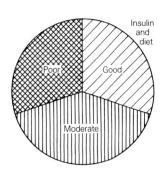

- good – 30%
- moderate – 40%
- poor – 30%

**long term care and
management**

resources available

- patient and his family
- GP and primary health care team
- hospital specialties

patient and family

education of the patient and his family is all-important

- clear and simple knowledge of diabetes and its complications
- follow appropriate diet
- self-monitoring urine/blood sugar and recording
- insulin techniques

    dose measurement

    injection technique

    care of syringes

- recognition and treatment of hypoglycaemia
- simple foot care

    hygiene

    well-fitting shoes

    attention to infections

    care with cutting toenails

GP and primary health care team

requirements

- medical assessment and advice
- dietary advice
- laboratory service for blood sugar
- chiropody service

regular follow-up to record

- diabetic symptoms – thirst, polyuria, loss of weight
- hypoglycaemic attacks
- cardiovascular – angina, breathlessness, claudication
- neurological – paraesthesiae, weakness
- eye problems
- foot problems

review patients' self-monitoring record

examine

- heart and peripheral arteries
- neurological signs legs
- fundi for retinopathy
- foot lesions

check

- urine
- blood sugar

hospital specialties

requirements

- diabetologist
- surgeon for peripheral vascular disease
- ophthalmologist for retinopathy
- obstetrician for pregnancy
- paediatrician for diabetic children

reserved for

- IDDM (Type I) difficult to control
- long term complications

N.B. diabetic nursing sister desirable as liaison between primary and secondary health care services

special problems

hypoglycaemia

- mainly in Type I (IDDM)
- causes
    delayed meal
    unusual exertion
    wrong dose of insulin
    accidental i.v. injection (rare)

- symptoms

    sweating

    shakiness

    apprehension

    palpitations

    pallor

    mental confusion

- if autonomic neuropathy present (or beta-blocker treatment) warning symptoms may be reduced or absent

- treatment

    patient himself – sugar lump, glucose tablet

    relative – 1 mg i.m. glucagon

    doctor – 20 ml 10% glucose i.v. stat

      long term – adjust insulin regimen

diabetic ketosis

- mortality

    5–10% in good centres

    50% in geriatric patients

- causes

    infections

    omitting dose of insulin

    mistaken (lower) dose of insulin

    heart attack/stroke/other trauma

- symptoms

    early – fatigue, thirst, polyuria, loss of weight

    late – vomiting, abdominal pain, leg cramps

- signs

    dehydration → dry skin, tongue

    air hunger → acetone smell on breath

    low blood pressure → weak rapid pulse

    abdominal tenderness and rigidity

    drowsiness and coma

- tests

    urine → heavy sugar, ketones

    blood → high sugar

    Na and K variable

    bicarbonate reduced, pH low

    high urea

- treatment   i.v. saline – up to 5 litres/24 h

    i.v. insulin – 5–6 units/h

    i.v. potassium – 20 mmol/h
    (monitor K level in blood)

    antibiotics

    nasogastric tube for aspiration

non-ketotic coma

hyperosmolar hyperglycaemic non-ketotic coma

- 5–10% of hyperglycaemic comas
- usually in elderly
- tests

    blood sugar > 50 mmol/l

    serum Na > 150 mmol/l

    plasma osmolality > 360 mmol/l

- treatment

    i.v. ½ normal saline for dehydration

    insulin i.v. as for ketoacidosis

    heparin i.v. to prevent disseminated
    intravascular coagulation

brittle diabetes (IDDM)

- mainly in young diabetics, especially girls
- possible causes

    poor dietary compliance

    irregular lifestyle

    faulty injection technique

    recurrent infection

    emotional stress

    hypoglycaemia with rebound hyperglycaemia (Somogyi effect)

- treatment

    rigorous home monitoring blood sugar

    multiple injections insulin

    may need i.m. rather than s.c. injections

    improvement home background

    psychotherapy

surgery

NIDDM

- omit oral drug if meals to be missed
- close monitoring blood sugar
- temporary insulin if sugar increases

IDDM

- continue usual insulin dose
- i.v. 5% dextrose
- supplement with i.v. insulin (0.5 – 2.0 units/h) if uncontrolled
- strict blood sugar control post-op to encourage wound healing

Useful practical points

- always think of diabetes in young patients with recurrent boils and in old patients with cataracts or unexplained loss of weight

- glycosuria may be a poor indication of either the presence of diabetes, especially in the elderly who may have a high renal threshold, or of the efficacy of diabetic control

- ketonuria indicates that insulin treatment is necessary in a diabetic

- regular supervision of the diabetic should always include assessment of the feet (for ischaemic and/or neuropathic disease), eyes (for retinopathy) and heart (for ischaemic disease)

- if a diabetic patient develops diarrhoea, especially at night, remember the complication of autonomic neuropathy

- it is important to diagnose proliferative retinopathy as soon as possible since treatment by laser photocoagulation will considerably reduce the loss of vision which usually results

14   EPILEPSY

WHAT IS IT?

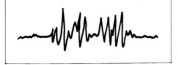

Figure 14.1   *e.e.g. showing paroxysmal spike discharge in epilepsy*

- paroxysmal/recurring fits or seizures
- produced by sudden excessive disorderly electrical discharges from brain cells – position, duration and site influence pattern of attack
- a 'symptom' and not a distinct disease – many possible causes but most attacks are idiopathic
- classification of epilepsy – this is based on that suggested by the Commission on classification of the terminology of epilepsy[37]

types

generalized seizures

- absence

  classic petit mal (3 per second spike and wave on e.e.g.)

  atypical

- myoclonic jerks (including salaams)
- grand mal with tonic/classic spasm
- akinetic

partial/focal

- simple (no impairment of consciousness)

  motor

  sensory

  autonomic

- complex (with impairment of consciousness)

  simple – followed by impaired consciousness

  impaired consciousness at onset

- partial evolving to grand mal

causes

infancy (0–1)

- congenital maldevelopment
    cortical dysplasia
    leukodystrophy
- birth injury/asphyxia
- infection
    congenital toxoplasmosis
    meningoencephalitis
- kernicterus
- phenylketonuria
- metabolic
    hypoglycaemia
    hypocalcaemia

childhood

- idiopathic
- febrile convulsions
- infection
    meningitis
    encephalitis
    brain abscess
- cerebral palsy, birth injury, perinatal anoxia
- congenital and degenerative
    tuberose sclerosis (epiloia)
    lipoidoses, e.g. Gaucher, Pick
    von Recklinghausen's disease
    Sturge–Weber disease
    galactosaemia
    aminoacidopathies
- Reye's syndrome – hepatic encephalopathy of unknown origin
- metabolic disorders – as above

adult

- idiopathic
- post-traumatic
- brain tumours (occur at all ages)
  - primary
  - secondary, especially cancer of lung
- vascular
  - cerebral infarct → atrophy
  - arteriovenous malformation
  - subdural haematoma
- infections
  - meningoencephalitis
  - brain abscess
  - syphilis
  - cysticercosis
  - toxoplasmosis
- metabolic
  - uraemic encephalopathy
  - hepatic encephalopathy
  - hypoglycaemia   spontaneous
  -                   insulin-induced in diabetics
  - hypocalcaemia, e.g. hypoparathyroidism
  - hypomagnesaemia
  - dialysis (aluminium intoxication)
- toxic
  - psychotropic drugs, e.g. tricyclic antidepressives
  - lead poisoning
  - lignocaine
  - aminophylline
- drug withdrawal
  - alcohol
  - sedatives, especially barbiturates

- dementia (some types)

  Huntington's chorea

  Jakob–Creutzfeldt disease

  Alzheimer's disease (rare)

N.B. In children and adults most epilepsy is 'idiopathic'

WHO GETS IT AND WHEN?

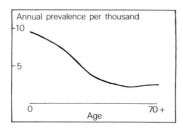

- epilepsy occurs at all ages but convulsive attacks are most prevalent in childhood

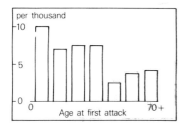

- epilepsy can commence at any age, but if febrile convulsions are included then most commence in childhood
- equal distribution in sexes

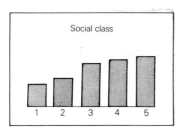

- higher prevalence in lower social groups

general practice

epilepsy in a practice population of 2500

Annual incidence of new cases	1–2
Annual prevalence of patients consulting	12–15
Cases with present or past epilepsy	50

district general hospital	DGH serving 250 000	
	Total cases of epilepsy (under treatment) in district	1250
	Attending hospital outpatient departments	250
	Admitted to hospital (including emergencies)	500

distribution of adult epilepsy

- 20% _generalized_   grand mal

                                   petit mal

                                   myoclonic

- 70% _partial_   15% simple

                                   40% complex

                                   10% partial → general

- 10% _unclassifiable_

WHAT HAPPENS?: NATURAL HISTORY/OUTCOMES OF IDIOPATHIC EPILEPSY

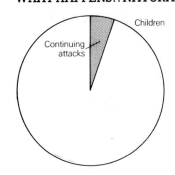

- _children (onset)_

     95% of all seizures will cease

     only one in 20 will go on to adult epilepsy

     only one in 100 will need special care and education

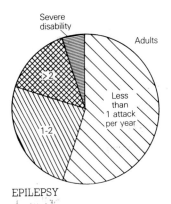

- _adults (onset)_

     55% will have less than one attack a year (many no attacks for 3 years+)

     30% – one to two attacks per year

     15% – more than two attacks per year

     5% – are seriously disabled

WHAT TO DO?

issues

- epileptic convulsions/seizures are terrifying for the lay person and worrying for the physician
- problems of diagnosis in excluding possible primary causes
- problems of long term control and personal, family, and social care and support
- prevention is possible by good obstetrics and good care of head injuries and c.n.s. infections
- specific cures possible in few
- all cases should be investigated neurologically in first instance
- long term care by general practitioner

DIAGNOSIS

clinical features of the various types

grand mal

- aura

  vague ascending abdominal discomfort

  feeling of apprehension

  olfactory – bad smells

  auditory – bells ringing

  visual – alteration form/shape

  hallucinations

- cry
- loss of consciousness
- tonic spasm

  tongue biting

  incontinence

- clonic spasms
- after-effects – headache

  confusion

  drowsiness

  automatism (rare)

absence	• classic *petit mal* only if accompanied by typical 3 per second spike and wave discharge on electroencephalogram
	• transient, very brief (5–10 s) alteration in consciousness
	sudden blankness
	sudden stare
	stops talking 5–10 secs
myoclonic jerks	• sudden brief episode of generalized muscle twitching not associated with alteration in consciousness
	• may produce a 'salaam' if twitching leads to flexion of trunk on hips
akinetic epilepsy	• sudden transient generalized loss of muscle tone
	• may result in sudden fall
	• immediate recovery
partial (focal) seizures	• the presentation will depend on the site of the epileptogenic focus
	• *partial motor* (Jacksonian)
	focus often starts in hand area of motor cortex (Figure 14.2)
	starts with twitching of thumb and index finger, spreads up arm to same side of face
	if discharge spreads across to opposite cortex →
	loss of consciousness
	generalized convulsion
	may be followed by transient residual monoparesis (Todd's paralysis)

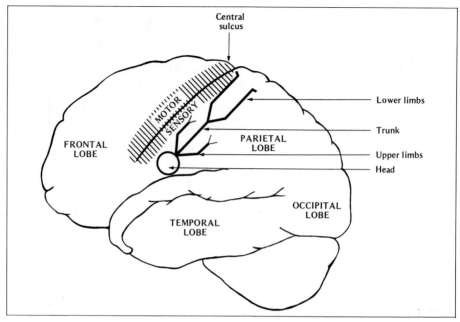

Figure 14.2 *Body representation in cerebral cortex*

- *partial sensory*

  similar pattern to Jacksonian epilepsy with a march of parasthesiae from the tip of a limb up to the trunk and face

- *partial autonomic*

  epigastric sensation

  pallor/flushing

  hair standing on end (piloerection)

  pupillary dilatation

- *psychomotor* (simple/complex partial seizure)

  originates in temporal lobe most frequently but also in frontal and occipital lobes

  symptoms

  déjà-vu phenomenon

  intense emotion

  unusual smells

  lip-smacking

  objects vary from small to large

  formed sensory hallucinations

  aimless behaviour

  automatic behaviour – may appear purposeful/skilful

- *febrile convulsions*

  children $^{6}/_{12}$–5 years, peak $^{9}/_{12}$–$^{20}/_{12}$

  seizure threshold reduced by fever

  occur in 3% all children

  tend to be familial

  usually single motor seizure

  e.e.g. is normal after seizure

  prognosis

  95% cease after 5 years with no subsequent epilepsy

  adverse features

  seizure > 15 min duration

  girl < 1½ years old

  boy < 2 years old

  pre-existing neurological abnormality

  frequent prolonged seizures

N.B. It is important to distinguish the benign febrile convulsion from the severe prolonged seizures associated with encephalitis

diagnosis of epilepsy

history

seizure

- complete and accurate description desirable
- often not obtainable from patient
- always speak to reliable observer if possible
- enquire about

  aura

  loss or alteration of consciousness

  tongue biting

  incontinence

  post-ictal headache

  post-ictal bizarre behaviour

general

- family history of epilepsy
- previous head trauma/birth trauma in infants/children
- cerebrovascular disease, e.g. stroke
- cardiovascular disease which may have led to a stroke

  heart attack

  cardiac arrhythmia

  rheumatic heart disease

- previous carcinoma treatment, e.g. breast, lung
- alcoholism
- drugs

  psychotropic, e.g. tricyclics

  barbiturates – withdrawal can precipitate epilepsy

- hypoglycaemia

  primary

    functional

    insulinoma

  secondary to insulin or hypoglycaemic
  drugs in diabetic

examination

the examination should be particularly
directed to

- evidence of cerebrovascular disease
- evidence of cardiovascular disease
- neurological disease

  focal signs

  raised intracranial pressure

  intracranial bruits

- evidence of malignancy

  breast

  lung

  enlarged glands

  enlarged liver

  abdominal mass

- evidence of liver disease
- evidence of kidney disease
- evidence of alcoholism

possible findings are shown in Figure 14.3

differential diagnosis of epilepsy

children

- breath holding attacks

  precipitating event

  usually cyanosed

  transient loss of consciousness

  loss of tone/increase tone

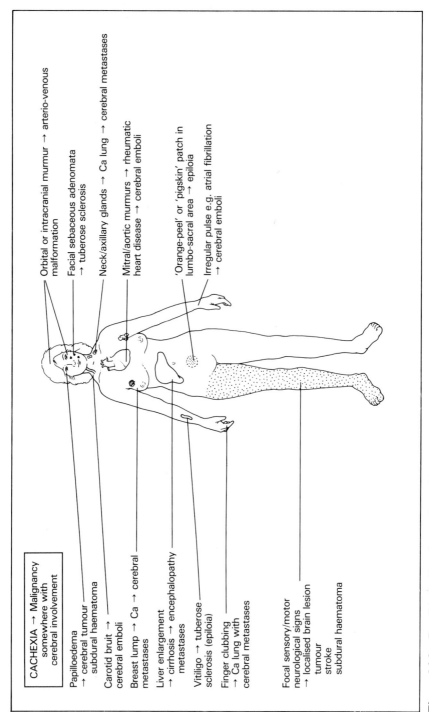

Figure 14.3 *Possible findings in a patient with epilepsy*

CACHEXIA → Malignancy somewhere with cerebral involvement

Papilloedema
→ cerebral tumour
subdural haematoma

Carotid bruit →
cerebral emboli

Breast lump → Ca → cerebral metastases

Liver enlargement
→ cirrhosis → encephalopathy
metastases

Vitiligo → tuberose sclerosis (epiloia)

Finger clubbing
→ Ca lung with cerebral metastases

Focal sensory/motor
neurological signs
→ localised brain lesion
tumour
stroke
subdural haematoma

Orbital or intracranial murmur → arterio-venous malformation

Facial sebaceous adenomata
→ tuberose sclerosis

Neck/axillary glands → Ca lung → cerebral metastases

Mitral/aortic murmurs → rheumatic heart disease → cerebral emboli

'Orange-peel' or 'pigskin' patch in lumbo-sacral area → epiloia

Irregular pulse e.g. atrial fibrillation
→ cerebral emboli

- syncopal attack

  micturition

  laryngeal

  postural

  reflex, e.g. venepuncture

N.B. may be associated with short tonic/clonic episode

- pseudoseizure

  usually adolescents

  may have true epilepsy also

  often family history of epilepsy

  'unconvincing' attacks

  usually when someone nearby

  no tongue biting/incontinence

  may last excessive time

- cardiac arrhythmia

  rare

  check e.c.g./ambulatory monitoring

- nightmares/night terrors

- daydreaming

  may be confused with petit mal

  child always 'accessible' during attack

  may be depressed child

- tics – may resemble myoclonic jerks

- cataplexy

  part of narcolepsy syndrome

  abnormal sleep attacks in day

  complete loss of tone 5–30 min

  often caused by emotional shock

adults

- syncope
    - gradual onset
    - nausea/sweating/fading vision
    - extreme pallor
    - rapid recovery on lying flat
    - occasional twitching/incontinence
    - may be preceded by
        - strong emotion
        - prolonged standing
        - vigorous exercise
        - micturition (often at night)
        - prolonged coughing
- arrhythmia
    - atrial fibrillation → palpitations
    - Stokes–Adams attack
        - previous angina/heart attack
        - sudden loss of consciousness
        - cyanosis
        - stertorous breathing
        - very slow or absent pulse
        - e.c.g. will decide (Figure 14.4)

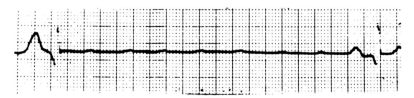

Figure 14.4   *e.c.g. showing P waves and no QRS in a Stokes–Adams attack*

- transient ischaemic attack (TIA)

  fully conscious patient

  convulsions very rare

  drop attack – no loss of consciousness

  brain stem symptoms   dysarthria

                        diplopia

                        dysphagia

  origin may be evident   carotid artery

                        arrhythmia

                        heart murmur

- hypoglycaemia

  may be a diabetic on treatment

  fits before breakfast or after prolonged fast

  other symptoms   sweating

                   palpitations

                   tremors

                   weakness

                   feeling of hunger

- narcolepsy – as in children

- migraine

  may produce focal symptoms and e.e.g. may be abnormal

  consciousness preserved

  vascular (throbbing) headache frequent

  family history of migraine

- psychogenic

  often occurs under emotional stress

  bizarre pattern of attack/behaviour

  rarely occurs in absence of witness

  no tongue biting/incontinence

- paroxysmal vertigo, e.g. Menière's disease

  associated tinnitus in attack

  deafness on examination

  audiometry will help in diagnosis

- hyperventilation
  - anxious individual – often adolescent girls
  - associated tingling in extremities
  - carpopedal spasm may occur
  - rapid recovery on rebreathing into paper or polythene bag

INVESTIGATIONS

electroencephalogram (e.e.g.)

objectives
- to confirm a diagnosis of epilepsy
- to establish the type for medication
- to indicate a cause, e.g. tumour

expected positive

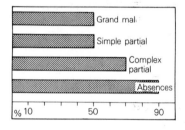

- grand mal epilepsy: 25–50%
- simple partial seizure: 50%
- complex partial seizure: 50–70%
- absences: 80–90%

types of abnormality
- epilepsy
  - grand mal – diffuse high voltage spikes
  - partial seizure – paroxysm of focal spike discharge (Figure 14.5)

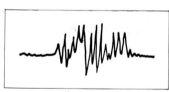

Figure 14.5 *Paroxysmal spike discharge (grand mal)*

classic petit mal – 3 per second spike and wave (Figure 14.6)

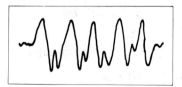

Figure 14.6 *3 per second spike and wave in petit mal*

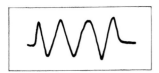

Figure 14.7 *Delta waves in brain tumour*

• tumour – focal slow (delta) wave (Figure 14.7)

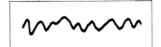

Figure 14.8 *Slow activity in cerebrovascular disease*

• cerebrovascular disease – widespread slow wave activity (Figure 14.8)

• brain injury – diffuse/focal slow wave activity
• hepatic encephalopathy – bilateral large triphasic waves (Figure 14.9)

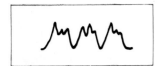

Figure 14.9 *Triphasic waves in hepatic coma*

• uraemic encephalopathy – bilateral high amplitude delta waves

other relevant points

• a positive e.e.g. is *not* necessary for a diagnosis of epilepsy
• the e.e.g. is more likely to be abnormal during or soon after the epileptic attack
• an abnormal e.e.g. may be produced in an epileptic by

    flashing light stimulation

    hyperventilation

    stimulant drug, e.g. leptazol

computerized axial tomography (CT scan) (Figure 14.10)

- best test for structural lesions (20% of epileptics overall)

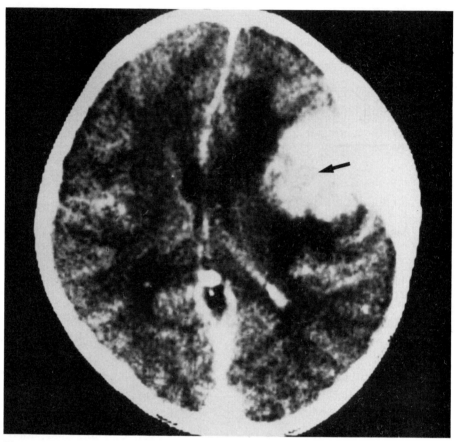

Figure 14.10 *CT scan showing a brain tumour (arrowed) – meningioma*

- recent onset epilepsy in an adult especially with focal neurological signs is main indication
- other indications

    seizures difficult to control – may show focal origin susceptible to surgery

    seizures changing in pattern – may indicate tumour

possible CT findings in epilepsy	• brain tumour
	• cerebral infarction
	• vascular malformations
	• hydrocephalus
	• calcification
	• congenital abnormalities

skull X-ray	• may show evidence of tumour
	• displacement of calcified pineal
	• calcification, e.g. meningioma
	• enlarged vascular channels, e.g. angioma
	• bone erosion – secondary carcinoma
	• increased bone density – meningioma

N.B. If a CT scan is available skull X-ray is superfluous

| **chest X-ray** | • for cancer of lung (with cerebral metastases) |

tests in symptomatic (secondary) epilepsy

- blood sugar – hypoglycaemia
- blood urea – uraemic encephalopathy
- blood ammonia – hepatic encephalopathy
- serum calcium – hypocalcaemia

MANAGEMENT OF EPILEPSY

general measures

education	• epilepsy is non-specific condition
	• there is no brain disease
	• anyone can become epileptic
	low blood sugar
	shortage of oxygen
	stimulant drugs

- fits can be controlled
- only slight chance of passing it on

work

- encourage normal work if possible
- avoid work where a seizure would be a danger to the patient or others
- not accepted in police, teaching, nursing

driving

- licence available if no attacks 3 years
- permitted if attacks only in sleep in the 3-year period
- cannot hold HGV or PSV licence

home

- fires well-guarded
- gates at top of stairs
- epileptic mother can bath baby if someone else present

schoolchildren

- minimum restrictions
- participate in all school activities
- swimming permitted if supervised

pregnancy

- may increase or reduce seizures
- avoid anticonvulsant in first 6–8 weeks if possible, especially phenytoin and valproate → fetal abnormality

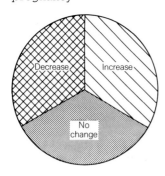

symptomatic treatment of seizures

aims
- to prevent seizures
- to avoid side-effects

principles
- get to know a few drugs well
- use one drug only if possible
- increase the dose progressively but slowly up to maximum permitted unless side-effects occur
- monitor blood level for

  therapeutic level

  toxic level
- select appropriate drug for type of seizure

Seizure	Drug	Adult dose
Grand mal	phenytoin (Epanutin)	150–300 mg b.d.
	sodium valproate (Epilim)	200–800 mg t.d.s.
	phenobarbitone (Luminal)	30–60 mg t.d.s.
	primidone (Mysoline)	250 mg t.d.s.
Petit mal	*classic* – ethosuximide (Zarontin)	0.5–2 g daily
	atypical –	
	sodium valproate (Epilim)	200–800mg t.d.s.
	clonazepam (Rivotril)	4–8 mg daily
Grand mal + petit mal	phenytoin (Epanutin)	150–300 mg bd
	sodium valproate (Epilim)	200–800 mg t.d.s.
	phenobarbitone (Luminal)	30–60 mg t.d.s.
Partial seizures	carbamazepine (Tegretol)	100–600 mg b.d.
	phenytoin (Epanutin)	150–300 mg b.d.
	primidone (Mysoline)	250–500 mg t.d.s.
	phenobarbitone (Luminal)	30–60 mg t.d.s.

N.B. Make an appropriate adjustment of dose for children

side-effects of anticonvulsants
- excessive sedation   phenobarbitone

  primidone
- rashes   phenobarbitone

  phenytoin
- alopecia   sodium valproate
- gingival hyperplasia   phenytoin

- ataxia   phenobarbitone

  phenytoin

  carbamazepine
- macrocytic anaemia   phenobarbitone

  phenytoin
- fetal abnormality   phenytoin

  sodium valproate
- hirsutism   phenytoin
- beware of drug interactions with phenytoin
  - → increased blood levels   diazepam

    chlorpromazine

    chlordiazepoxide

    imipramine

    sulphonamides

    chloramphenicol
  - → reduced blood levels   antacids

    isoniazide

    chlorpheniramine

status epilepticus

- continuous generalized convulsions
- frequent recurrent convulsions with no recovery of consciousness between attacks
- precipitating factors

  withdrawal of anticonvulsants

  failure to take treatment for epilepsy

  brain trauma

  acute infections

  brain tumour

  metabolic disturbances   sodium

                                          potassium

                                          calcium

                                          sugar

  uraemia

- dangers

hypoxia
hyperpyrexia
hypoglycaemia
acidosis
$\left.\right\}$ → permanent brain damage

management

- emergency admission to hospital
- intravenous infusion
- blood samples for   sugar
  electrolytes
  pH and blood gases
  anticonvulsant drug levels
- drugs

  1st line

  diazepam 10–15 mg i.v. in 1–2 min repeat with each fit up to total 50 mg

  phenytoin 1–1.5 g at rate of 50 mg/min

  2nd line

  if seizures continue > 30 min

  phenobarbitone 1–1.5 g i.v. at no more than 25 mg/min

  3rd line

  after 60 min

  i.v. paraldehyde 0.1 mg/in 5–10 ml of saline

  i.v. lignocaine 50–100 mg

  i.v. lorazepam 0.05–0.15 mg/kg at 1 mg/min up to 8 mg

  if still resistant – i.v. thiopentone anaesthesia and be prepared for ventilatory support

Useful practical points

- epilepsy is a symptom
- try and discover the cause
- three quarters are idiopathic
- epilepsy is a serious personal/family situation
- good prognosis
- good control of fits possible
- severe mental/physical disability in a small minority only
- use as few drugs as possible but more than one may be necessary in difficult cases
- an abnormal e.e.g. is not necessary to confirm epilepsy – it is a *clinical* diagnosis
- a child or young adult with a single seizure and no physical signs requires neither investigation nor treatment
- a recent focal fit in an adult, especially with focal neurological signs, should always be considered a brain tumour until proven otherwise

15   MULTIPLE SCLEROSIS

WHAT IS IT?

- a disease of unknown aetiology characterized pathologically by patches of demyelination in the central nervous system
- the demyelination is disseminated in space (in the nervous system) and in time leading to focal neurological defects. There are certain sites of predilection

    cervical cord

    optic nerves

    periventricular

- it is the commonest disabling disease of young adults in the United Kingdom
- the cause is unknown but the factors which may be involved are

    altered immunological reaction in the nervous system

    infectious agent – some support from epidemiological studies, e.g. occupation of the Faroes (no previous cases of MS) by British troops – cases of MS followed

    environmental factor – different incidence in different parts of the world

- the most popular current theory of aetiology is a slowly-developing altered immunological reaction in the central nervous system in response to an infection, probably a virus, early in life

- there are some well-established precipitating factors

  infections with pyrexia

  physical trauma, e.g. operation

  emotional shocks

  pregnancy

  changes of temperature

WHO GETS IT AND WHEN?

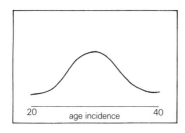

- a disease of young adults

  20–40 years

  peak 30 years

  $F : M = 3 : 2$

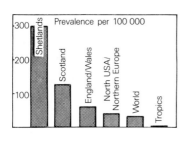

- prevalence

  World   30/100 000

  England/Wales   50–80/100 000

  Scotland   125/100 000

  Shetlands   300/100 000

  North USA/Northern Europe   30–80/100 000

  Tropics   < 1/100 000

- may occur in families – the risk in a first degree relative is 15 × the general population.

- migration from an area of low incidence to one of high incidence will only alter the risk if migration occurs in childhood[39]

| frequency (in UK) | • annual incidence (new cases) : ten per 100 000 |
| | • point prevalence : 75 per 100 000 |

general practice

multiple sclerosis in population of 2500

New cases	1 every 5 years
In practice	2–3
(Severe	1–2)

district general hospital

DGH serving 250 000

Annual admissions (for MS)	30
MS in DGH area	250
(Severely disabled	175)

WHAT HAPPENS?

multiple sclerosis is unpredictable in its course and outcome

course and prognosis

- relapse rate 0.3–0.4 attacks/year per 100[40]

    < 1 year in 30%

    < 2 years in another 20%

    5–9 years in a further 20%

    10–30 years another 10%

- 10% – steadily progressive disease
- average lifespan > 20 years
- after 25 years

    one third patients still working

    two thirds still ambulatory[41]

- one sixth have benign course 10–15 years, then become severe
- one sixth only slight disability 15 years from onset
- one third die within 20 years

prognostic features

good
- onset < 40 years age
- onset with sensory symptoms
- onset with retrobulbar neuritis
- long interval between 1st → 2nd attacks
- infrequent relapses

bad
- onset > 40 years age
- onset with brainstem involvement
- < 1 year between 1st and 2nd attacks
- frequent relapses

possible courses

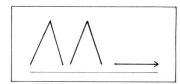

- abrupt onset
  few, if any relapses
  no residual disability

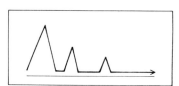

- relapses of diminishing frequency and severity
  slight disability

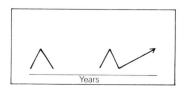

- abrupt onset
  long period of remission
  slow progression

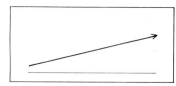

- slow relentless progression from onset

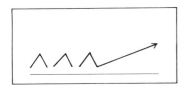

- recurrent frequent relapses with progression

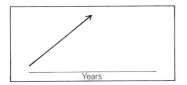

- severe rapid deterioration and early death

likely outcomes (over 20 years)

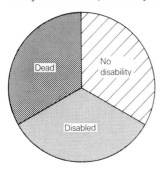

- one third – slight or no disability
- one third – moderate/severe disability
- one third – dead

mortality

- in about 5% progressive and rapid death
- in majority life expectancy is 25 years + from time of diagnosis

clinical features

history

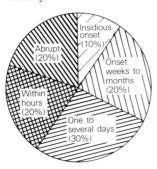

- onset may be
  - within minutes
  - within hours
  - within days
  - within weeks/months
  - slow steady progression
- 80% present with one symptom only

initial symptoms	<ul><li>weakness/numbness in limbs (50%)</li><li>retrobulbar neuritis (25%)</li><li>others in descending frequency
	    unsteady walking
	    brainstem diplopia
	                     vertigo
	                     vomiting
	    disorders of micturition</li><li>less common manifestations
	    trigeminal neuralgia
	    facial paralysis
	    hemiplegia/dysphasia/hemianaesthesia
	    fits
	    euphoria
	    leg and girdle pains</li></ul>

limb weakness	<ul><li>*lower limbs > upper limbs*</li><li>shows as
	    heaviness
	    stiffness
	    weakness
	    tiredness
	    tendency to trip
	    catching toe in carpet
	    sudden giving way</li><li>may only show after
	    heavy exertion
	    hot bath</li><li>symptoms may occur in one leg but signs almost always in both</li></ul>

sensory symptoms	<ul><li>usually affects lower limbs and trunk</li><li>numbness (tingling) begins in one or both feet and spreads upwards to trunk/waist over several days</li><li>sensory symptom may remain localized to one limb or to the face</li><li>posterior column involvement may lead to</li></ul>

sensory symptoms

- usually affects lower limbs and trunk
- numbness (tingling) begins in one or both feet and spreads upwards to trunk/waist over several days
- sensory symptom may remain localized to one limb or to the face
- posterior column involvement may lead to

  'useless hand' – power normal but coordination gone

  unsteady walking on wide base with high-stepping gait

  bizarre leg symptoms, e.g. feels 'swollen' or 'missing'

- loss of sensation may involve

  urethra

  vagina

  rectum

- *Lhermitte's sign* – sensation of electric shock in back and limbs on flexing the neck – frequent in MS but actually first described by Babinski in cervical cord trauma

retrobulbar neuritis

- evolves over several hours to several days
- pain in eye (worse on moving eye) may precede visual disturbance by 1–2 days
- usually only one eye but sometimes other eye involved simultaneously or within few weeks
- visual disturbance

  may be transient blurring

  may be partial blindness

  may be total blindness

- recovery

  one third recover completely

  one third improve considerably

  one third little or no improvement

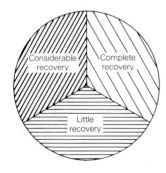

	• improvement starts within 2–3 weeks
	• 50% will develop other manifestations of multiple sclerosis within 15 years
ataxia	• leads to unsteadiness and incoordination
	• may be due to posterior column involvement with loss of joint/proprioceptive sense
	• may be due to cerebellar involvement leading to incoordination of voluntary movement, e.g.

ataxia

- leads to unsteadiness and incoordination
- may be due to posterior column involvement with loss of joint/proprioceptive sense
- may be due to cerebellar involvement leading to incoordination of voluntary movement, e.g.

    lifting a cup → spills

    walking → veering to one side

    inability to stand steady – due to truncal ataxia (plaque in tegmentum of midbrain)

    may affect speech → 'scanning' speech (every syllable pronounced)

- isolated cerebellar involvement is uncommon in MS

brain stem involvement

- diplopia

    due to involvement medial longitudinal bundle in the midbrain (Figure 15.1)

    weakness usually affects medial and lateral rectus muscles in both eyes

    diplopia occurs on lateral gaze

    impairment of conjugate deviation upwards may occur

- dysarthria – often associated with parasthesiae of the face and upper limbs (Figure 15.2)
- vertigo/vomiting – due to involvement of vestibular connections
- deafness/tinnitus – cochlear connections
- trigeminal neuralgia – always consider MS as possible cause in young patient
- facial paralysis/anaesthesia – rare

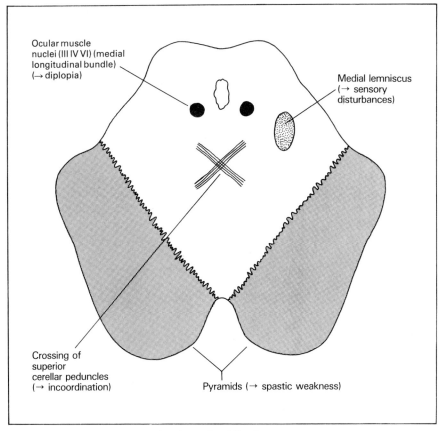

Figure 15.1 *Transverse section through midbrain*

N.B. when brainstem symptoms occur they may be associated with

- quadriplegia
- cerebellar ataxia
- pseudobulbar palsy

disorders of micturition

- occur in 10%
- symptoms

  hesitancy

  urgency

  frequency

  incontinence

- due to spinal cord involvement
- retention is rare
- in males, often associated with impotence (40–60%)

psychological disturbances
- euphoria – rare – due to frontal lobe lesion
- depression – probably result of the disease
- dementia – rare complication

examination
- some of the signs which may be found are shown in Figure 15.3
- Charcot's triad

nystagmus

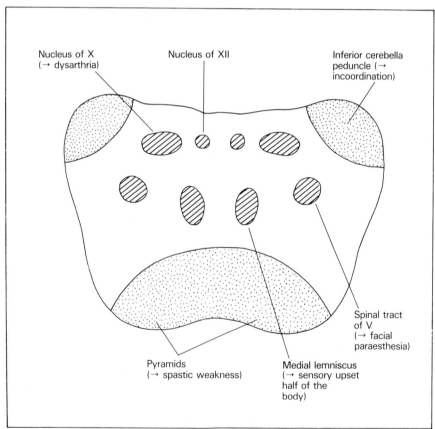

Figure 15.2 *Transverse section through the medulla*

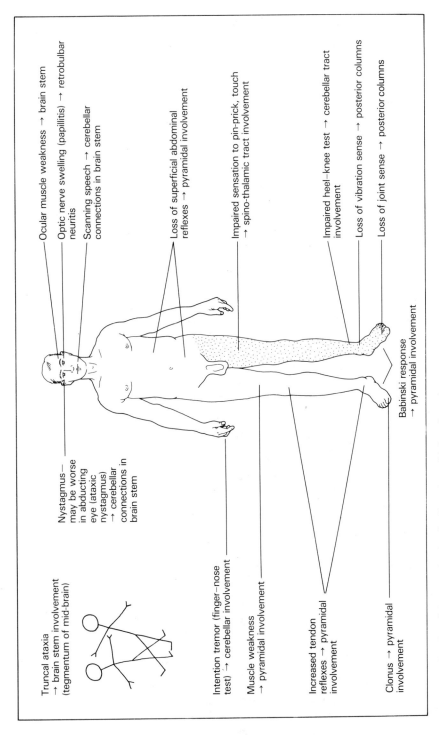

Figure 15.3 *Possible examination findings in multiple sclerosis*

Ocular muscle weakness → brain stem

Optic nerve swelling (papillitis) → retrobulbar neuritis

Scanning speech → cerebellar connections in brain stem

Loss of superficial abdominal reflexes → pyramidal involvement

Impaired sensation to pin-prick, touch → spino-thalamic tract involvement

Impaired heel–knee test → cerebellar tract involvement

Loss of vibration sense → posterior columns

Loss of joint sense → posterior columns

Babinski response → pyramidal involvement

Nystagmus— may be worse in abducting eye (ataxic nystagmus) → cerebellar connections in brain stem

Truncal ataxia → brain stem involvement (tegmentum of mid-brain)

Intention tremor (finger–nose test) → cerebellar involvement

Muscle weakness → pyramidal involvement

Increased tendon reflexes → pyramidal involvement

Clonus → pyramidal involvement

scanning speech

intention tremor

due to cerebellar tract involvement in brainstem

- established syndromes in longstanding disease

mixed (40%) – involvement

optic nerves

brain stem

cerebellum

spinal cord

spastic ataxia (30–40%) spinal involvement

pontocerebellar (5%)

impairment of vision (5%)

at 10–15 years the typical patient is shown in Figure 15.4

differential diagnosis

spinal cord compression

- pain over vertebra
- root pain
- pain worse on straining/coughing
- persistent cutaneous sensory level
- Brown–Séquard syndrome may be result (Figure 15.5)
- diagnostic test – myelogram

subacute combined degeneration of spinal cord – see Figure 15.6

distinguishing features

- anaemia – may be absent
- atrophic tongue
- test – serum B_{12} level will decide

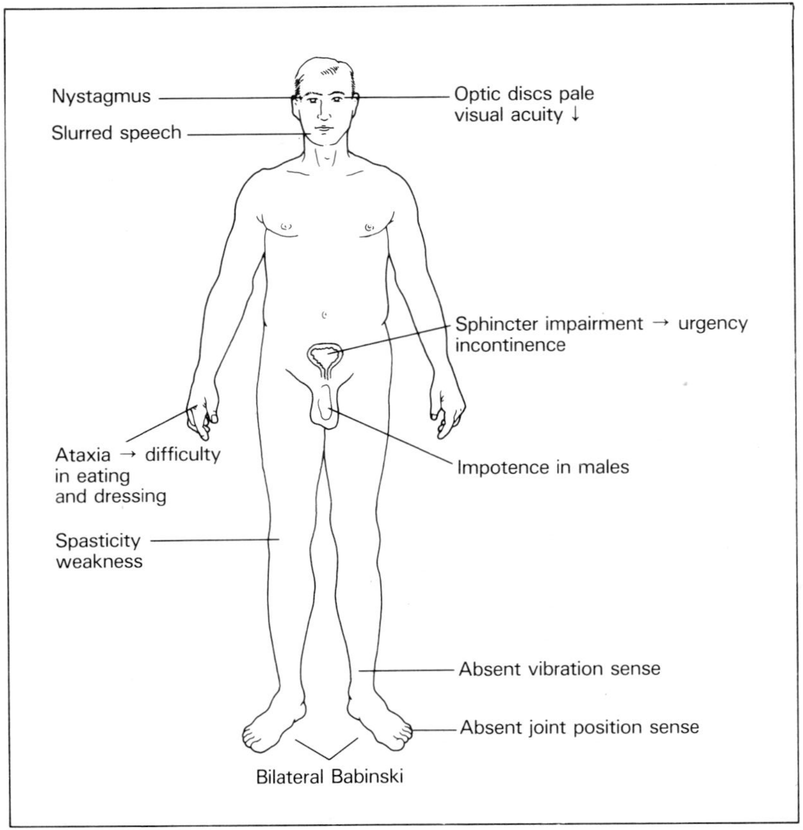

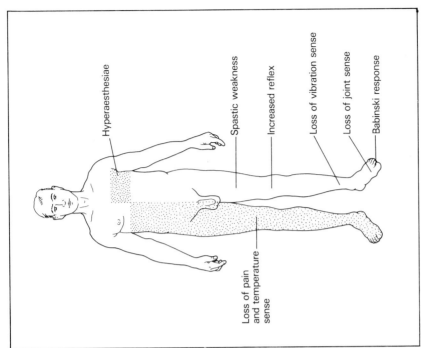

Figure 15.4 *Clinical features in long-established patient with MS*

Figure 15.5 *Brown–Séquard syndrome due to compression of half of the spinal cord*

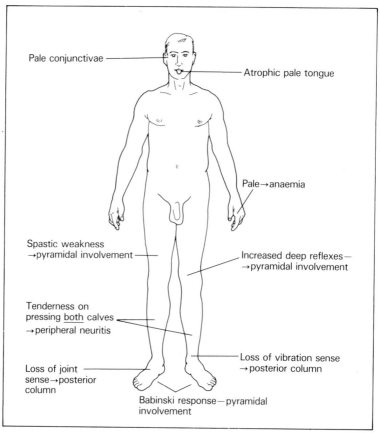

Pale conjunctivae

Atrophic pale tongue

Pale→anaemia

Spastic weakness
→pyramidal involvement

Increased deep reflexes—
→pyramidal involvement

Tenderness on
pressing both calves
→peripheral neuritis

Loss of vibration sense
→posterior column

Loss of joint
sense→posterior
column

Babinski response—pyramidal
involvement

Figure 15.6 *Subacute combined degeneration of the spinal cord*

hereditary spinocerebellar degeneration– see Figure 15.7

distinguishing features

- family history
- pes cavus and scoliosis
- conduction defects (e.c.g.)
- lack of remissions

hemiplegic type of MS

- cerebrovascular accident
- brain tumour
- test – CT scan will decide

MULTIPLE SCLEROSIS

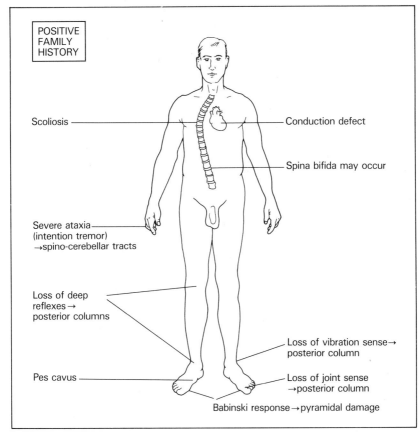

Figure 15.7 *Friedereich's ataxia*

collagen disease

- ESR high
- SLE – multisystem involvement
- polyarteritis nodosa
    collagen screen will help
    autoantibodies help

other rarer conditions

- sarcoidosis
- multiple emboli
- neurosyphilis
- Behçet's syndrome

investigations

- cerebrospinal fluid

    mild lymphocytosis 10–15 cells/mm^3

    mild protein increase 40–80 mg/100 ml

    increase in gammaglobulin

    Lange curve : paretic (first zone rise)

    negative test for syphilis

- visual – evoked reflex

    visual stimulation with a flashing light and measurement of response time in the occipital cortex with an electroencephalogram

    prolonged response time in MS > 115 msec

    other conditions can prolong

      glaucoma

      compression optic nerve

      degeneration optic nerve

- CT scan – may show a plaque

- nuclear magnetic resonance likely to be much more helpful

TREATMENT

three guiding principles

- sympathetic understanding – incurable, progressive, disabling and unpredictable disease

- control symptoms where possible

- be sceptical of new 'cures'

general

- physiotherapy

    strengthen alternative muscles

    maintain joint mobility

    prevent contractures

    improve coordination by exercises

    exercises to reduce spasticity

    swimming aids mobility

- avoid overfatigue at work or play
- control infection promptly to prevent relapse
- walking aids
    leg irons for foot-drop
    knee cage for hyperextensibility
    tetrapod
    walking frame
- wheelchair when necessary
    for home use
    for outdoor use
- bedbound patient
    treat respiratory infections
    treat urinary infections
    treat bedsores
    treat leg vein thrombosis
- psychological support
    understanding
    sympathy
    honesty
    optimism within the bounds of feasibility of symptom control
- support groups may help, e.g. MS Society
    improves knowledge of disease
    sharing of problems
    social events
    updates on research → optimistic outlook
    financial help for research
- *constipation*
    high fibre diet (fruit, leafy vegetables)
    bran products
    stool softener, e.g. liquid paraffin

- *impotence*
    - no specific treatment
    - testosterone no good
    - sex counsellor may help
- *trigeminal neuralgia*
    - phenytoin 100 mg t.d.s.
    - carbamazepine (Tegretol) 200–400 mg t.d.s.
    - neurosurgery – alcohol injection
        - nerve section

specific treatment

- the only treatment which has stood the test of time is steroid therapy
- it is only of value for an acute relapse of MS and of no value in long term prophylaxis
- ACTH used in UK – dosage
    - first week 60 units i.m. daily
    - second week 40 units i.m. daily
    - third week 20 units i.m. daily

side-effects must be considered

- fluid retention
    - weight gain (weigh daily)
    - oedema
    - hypertension
- hypokalaemia
    - common
    - use prophylactic K-retaining diuretic, e.g. triamterene or amiloride
- hyperglycaemia – not an important problem except in a diabetic patient
- mental disturbance
    - rare
    - tends to occur at end of or immediately after the course

symptomatic treatment

- *spasticity*

    baclofen (Lioresal)

        initially 5 mg t.d.s.

        maximum 100 mg daily

        dose critical

        overdose → flaccidity

    dantrolene (Dantrium)

        initially 25 mg/day

        maximum 100 mg q.d.s.

        occasionally causes chronic active
        hepatitis – so monitor liver function

    diazepam (Valium)

        initially 2–15 mg t.d.s.

        maximum 60 mg daily

    surgical measures available in severe cases

        phenol injection

        neurotomy

        tenotomy

        tendon transplant

- *urinary upsets*

retention	methyldopa	250 mg 1–2/day
	phenoxybenzamine	10 mg 1–2/day
incontinence	Pro-Banthine	7.5–15 mg 1–4/day
	Cetiprin	200 mg t.d.s.
urgency	ephedrine	15 mg 1–3/day
infection	antibiotic	

other treatment

many other treatments have been tried but there is no convincing evidence to date of any sustained or objective benefits:

- gluten-free diet
- diet high in polyunsaturated fatty acids

- cytotoxic agents e.g.

  azathioprine

  cyclophosphamide
- hyperbaric oxygen
- transfer factor treatment to improve immune responses
- intrathecal interferon
- spinal cord stimulation

Useful practical points

- retrobulbar neuritis associated with spinal cord symptoms is highly suspicious of multiple sclerosis
- hemiplegia is a rare presentation of multiple sclerosis – always consider stroke and brain tumour as possible causes first
- consider multiple sclerosis in any young patient presenting with features of trigeminal neuralgia
- onset of multiple sclerosis with retrobulbar neuritis carries a good prognosis
- onset over 45 years of age carries a bad prognosis
- steroid therapy is of no long term prophylactic value in multiple sclerosis
- a 3-week course of steroids can be tried with an acute relapse or if an adverse change in neurological function occurs, even if there is no clear-cut onset of the deterioration

---

16   MIGRAINE

WHAT IS IT?

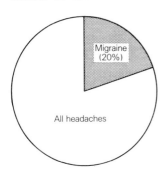

Migraine (20%)

All headaches

- 'Migraine' is a common label but precise diagnostic criteria are difficult to define
- migraine is a part of a much larger collection of headaches
- migraine probably makes up one fifth of all headaches
- the *syndrome* of *migraine* comprises all or some of

  episodic/paroxysmal unilateral headache

  nausea/vomiting

  prodromal aura – usually visual

  associated symptoms

  mood change

  fluid retention

  diuresis

  yawning

  sometimes transient neurological disturbances

classification

a *classification of migraine* (and there are many)

- common migraine = predominantly headache
- classical migraine = headache with nausea/vomiting
- complete migraine = headache, nausea/vomiting and prodromal aura
- migrainous neuralgia

- complicated migraine
  - hemiplegic
  - ophthalmoplegic
  - vertebrobasilar
- symptomatic migraine
  - a–v malformation
  - aneurysm
- migraine equivalents – prodromata without headache or vomiting – may predate classical migraine

pathophysiology of migraine

- intracranial vasoconstriction → aura
- extracranial vasodilation → headache
- release of
  - serotonin
  - kinins
  - catecholamines
- trigger factors
  - physical/mental stress
  - food allergy
    - cheese
    - chocolate
    - alcohol
  - hormonal changes, e.g. periods
- there is a *migraine* diathesis that involves certain individuals with certain personalities, social backgrounds and family histories

migraine diathesis

tense

social class 1 > 5

FH +

go-getter

WHO SUFFERS WHEN?

- 80% of the population suffer headaches in any year
- 20% of headaches are migraine
- $F > M = 2:1$
- community questionnaire surveys suggest that 20% of population suffer migraines (10 million in UK)
- in general practice 10% of population consult for migraine over a *10-year period* (5 million in UK)
- *annual* prevalence (consulting) rate in general practice is 2% (1 million)

Population profile of migraine

20% suffer migraine ever
(half consult GP ever)

10% consult GP ever

2% consult GP in a year

---

frequency

general practice

migraine in practice population of 2500: annual numbers

Persons suffering attacks	500
Persons consulting over 10 years	250
Annual prevalence of patients consulting	50
(Referred to hospital	1)
(Migrainous neuralgia	1–2)
(Complicated migraine	1 every 5 years)

district general hospital

DGH serving 250 000 persons

Migraine referrals to outpatient departments annual	100

age prevalence

- *onset* – migraine can start at any age but most begin to suffer attacks in teens or early adult life

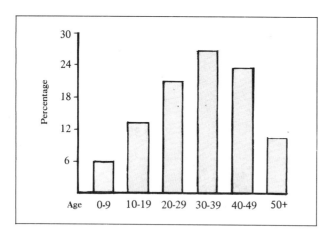

- *annual age prevalence*

  F > M

  peak 20–40 in F

  less of a peak in M

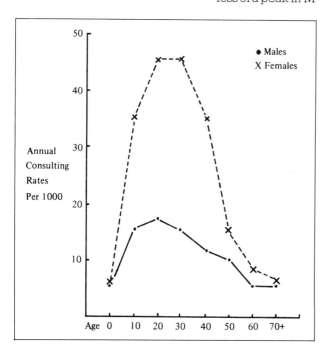

WHAT HAPPENS?

natural history

- in most there is a 'period of activity' during which attacks of migraine occur – this may be up to 20 years – followed by cessation of attacks

severity

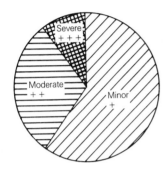

- during that time the grades of severity are likely to be

	% of migraine sufferers
Severe +++ severe and frequent with disruption of life	10%
Moderate ++ attacks at least once a month with inconvenience	30%
Minor + minor and a nuisance	60%

outcome

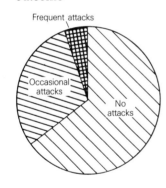

- after 20 years from onset

no attacks	65%
occasional attacks (1–2 per year)	30%
frequent attacks (at least one every 3 months)	5%

clinical features

typical attack

prodromata

- visual commonest fortification spectra
  - scintillations
  - scotomata
  - hemianopia
- sensory – paraesthesia/numbness start in upper limb → face
- weakness/dysphasia sometimes

headache

- usually unilateral
- not always on same side
- thumping/throbbing
- may last few hours to several days
- associated with photophobia
- coughing/sneezing/head movement exacerbates
- often followed by marked diuresis

nausea/vomiting

- starts after headache starts
- vomiting may terminate attack

trigger factors

- the most frequent factors are shown in Figure 16.1
- other factors
  - missed meals
  - insomnia
  - physical heat/cold
    - flashing lights
    - loud noise
  - excessive exercise
  - travelling (anxiety)
  - changing moods

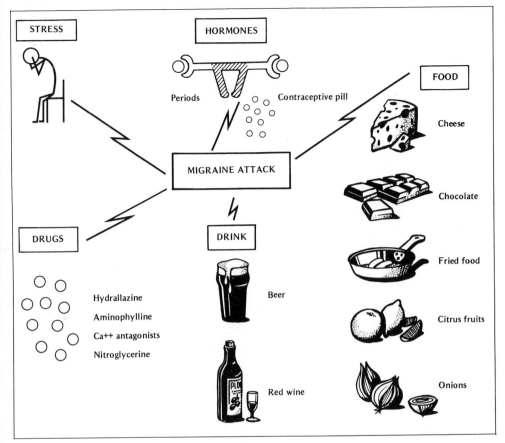

Figure 16.1 *Trigger factors in migraine*

special types of migraine

migrainous neuralgia (cluster headache)

- the typical clinical features are shown in Figure 16.2
- occasional manifestations

    flushing of face

    partial ptosis/miosis

- in between clusters of headache, patient may be free for months or years
- alcohol is a frequent precipitant even in very small amounts

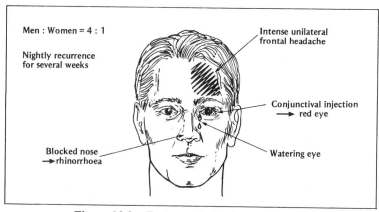

Men : Women = 4 : 1

Nightly recurrence
for several weeks

Intense unilateral
frontal headache

Conjunctival injection
→ red eye

Blocked nose
→rhinorrhoea

Watering eye

Figure 16.2 *Features of migrainous neuralgia*

complicated migraine

- hemiplegic

    unilateral limb weakness occurs during or
    after the headache and may last for several
    days

    strong familial tendency

- ophthalmoplegic

    associated with weakness of eye movement
    (involvement of 3rd cranial nerve)

    children usually affected

- vertebrobasilar

    prodromata due to ischaemia of brainstem

    vertigo

    double vision

    paraesthesiae

    unsteadiness

    transient loss of consciousness

    the headache tends to be occipital

migrainous equivalents

- *prodromata* of migraine without the
  subsequent headache and vomiting

- in children – *recurrent abdominal pain*

- in adults – *bilious attacks*

- may predate the development of classical
  migraine

permanent neurological damage

- rarely the neurological manifestations associated with migraine may become permanent

    hemianopia

    hemiplegia

- cerebral infarction may be found on CT scan
- the contraceptive pill may be a contributory factor

status migrainosus

- frequent attacks of migraine leaving the scalp continuously tender
- may be associated with constantly recurring focal neurological signs
- often precipitated by

    menopause

    development of hypertension

differential diagnosis

tension headache

- character

    pressure

    weight on head

    band round head

- site

    vertex mostly

    any other area

    often 'all over'

- lasts hours, days, weeks, months
- related to mental stress
- other anxiety symptoms

hypertensive headache

- throbbing
- occipital
- worse night/on waking
- severe hypertension

brain tumour

- throbbing/bursting
- worse at night/on waking
- worse coughing/straining
- nausea/vomiting which do *not* relieve the headache
- occipital → posterior fossa tumour
- frontoparietal → cerebral tumour

temporal arteritis

- temporal area – unilateral
- throbbing early – later aching or burning
- may be continuous weeks/months
- associated with   fever
    - loss of weight
    - muscle pains
    - loss of vision

depression

- non-specific headache may occur
- other symptoms of depression
    - anorexia
    - insomnia
    - early morning waking
    - can't concentrate
    - forgetfulness
    - fatigue
    - constipation
    - spells of weeping

cough headache

- middle-aged or elderly men
- headache provoked by
    - coughing
    - sneezing
    - straining

- frontal or occipital
- unilateral or bilateral
- bursting pain
- lasts few seconds to few minutes
- occasionally results from posterior fossa tumour

investigations   none usually required for classical migraine

indications
- onset in middle age
- focal neurological symptoms or signs
    hemiplegia
    ophthalmoplegia – especially if no family history
    status migrainosus
- if the headache in migraine is always unilateral

tests
- CT scan
    brain tumour
    angioma
    a–v malformation
- arteriography
    brain tumour   vascular
                           avascular
    vascular abnormality   angioma
                           a–v malformation
                           aneurysm

treatment

general measures
- patient education
    nature of condition
    benefits of treatment
    limitations of treatment

- avoidance of trigger factors
- avoidance stressful situations
- diuretic in premenstrual week
- discourage contraceptive pill or oestrogens for menopause
- avoid peripheral dilators, e.g. for hypertension

treatment of an attack

- *mild attack*

  simple analgesic early in attack

  aspirin

  paracetamol

  possibly an antiemetic, e.g. metoclopramide (Maxolon) 5–10 mg up to t.d.s.

- *severe attack*

  rest in darkened room

  ergot preparation

  oral

  suppository

  aerosol

  injection

  combined preparations – contain a mixture of ergot, analgesic and antiemetic, e.g. Migril, Migraleve

prophylactic treatment   *drugs*

- diazepam – 2 mg t.d.s.
- pizotifen (Sanomigran) 1.5–6.0 mg/day in divided doses
- clonidine (Dixarit) 50–70 mg b.d.
- methysergide (Deseril)

    1–2 mg t.d.s.

    short courses only

    danger of retroperitoneal fibrosis with prolonged treatment
- propranolol (Inderal) 40–80 mg t.d.s.

    other measures – relaxation therapy – claimed to help in 80%

Useful practical points

- the onset of migraine in a middle-aged patient should always raise the possibility of underlying organic disease
- migraine associated with paresis of the external ocular muscles may be due to an aneurysm on the posterior communicating artery of the circle of Willis
- don't forget to listen over the orbits and skull for a systolic murmur due to a–v malformation in any patient with late onset migraine – in practice this will be found very rarely
- in severe cases ergot preparations should be taken with the first symptoms of a migrainous headache – but the drug has no effect on the prodromata and may make them worse
- if vomiting does not relieve the headache in migraine, consider the possibility of brain tumour
- any change in the nature of the headache in longstanding migraine is suspicious of the development of alternative and potentially serious organic disease

17   PARKINSONISM

WHAT IS IT?

- a neurological disorder of largely unknown cause resulting from damage to or degeneration of basal ganglia (Figure 17.1)

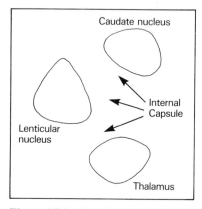

Figure 17.1   *Basal ganglia*

- caused by deficiency of the neurotransmitter dopamine
- characterized by slowness of movement, rigidity, tremor and ultimately mental deterioration

WHO GETS IT WHEN?

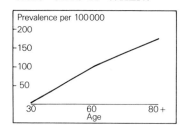

- a disorder associated with ageing
- M : F = 3 : 2
- whites > blacks

causes

- genetic factors may be important when condition present < 40 years old
- cerebral arteriosclerosis may be a cause (common)
- it may follow encephalitis in childhood (v. rare)
- autotoxins may cause premature neuronal death in idiopathic disease
- may be *less* frequent in cigarette smokers
- may follow use of drugs (see page 287)

• idiopathic (unknown cause)	75%
• arteriosclerotic	20%
• drug effects	5%
• post-encephalitic	1%

frequency

- *prevalence* in the community is 15 per 10 000
- 65% present in 50s and 60s
- in over-65s, over 10% of population have some features of parkinsonism[2]

general practice

parkinsonism in general practice with population of 2500

New case (incidence)	1 every 3 years
Annual prevalence (patients consulting)	4
Mortality	1 in 10 years

DGH serving population of 250 000	
Parkinson's disease patients in district	400 (half are severely affected)
New cases per year	35
Annual admissions	50
Attending OPD	250
Annual deaths	10

WHAT HAPPENS?

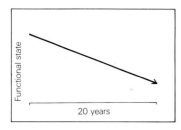

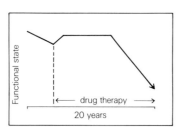

- progressive disorder with ultimate severe disability unless death intervenes from other cause
- duration of disease usually 10–20 years
- rates of deterioration are variable

  some rapid

  some slower

  in some deterioration may apparently stop
- modern drugs can delay deterioration and improve condition for some years (5–10) but then benefits tend to cease

clinical features

history

- insidious onset – may take several years
- *tremor* – commonest initial presentation (80%)

  hands primarily affected especially thumb

  later spread to   forearms

                        head and neck

                        tongue

                        lower limbs – least common

present at rest and improves with purposeful activity

may be worse under emotional stress

- *reduction of mobility (akinesia)*

    rising from a chair difficult

    walking and turning difficult

    writing – handwriting becomes smaller and less legible

    dressing/undressing slow

    feeding very slow

    speech affected   voice becomes soft

                          slow starting

                          difficulty in enunciating

                          monotonous

- *mental changes*

    depression common

    eventually dementia may occur (15–30%)

- *other symptoms*

    constipation

    excessive sweating

    increased salivation especially in post-encephalitic type

    weight loss

    bladder disturbances

examination   the findings are shown in Figure 17.2

differential diagnosis

physiological tremor (senile or 'essential' tremor)

- faster than parkinsonian tremor
- increased by anxiety
- occurs in one plane
- lacks 'pill-rolling' character
- worse on volitional movement
- lack of associated slowness of movement

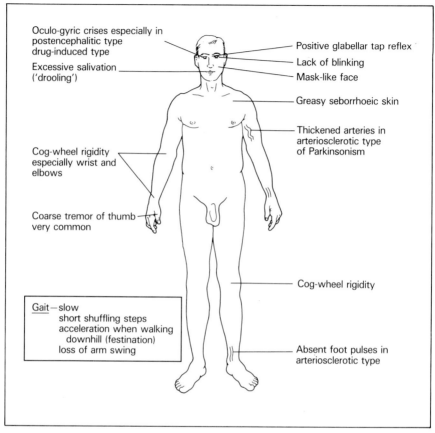

Figure 17.2 *Findings in Parkinson's disease*

- relieved by alcohol
- often familial

arteriosclerotic dementia
- stepwise progression
- pseudobulbar palsy may be present
  emotional lability
  dysarthria
  dysphagia
- pyramidal signs present
  increased jaw jerk
  increased reflexes
  extensor plantar responses

low-pressure hydrocephalus	● previous head injury
	meningitis
	subarachnoid haemorrhage
	● impairment of mental function
	● slowly progressive gait disorder
	● urinary/faecal incontinence

myxoedema

● mental and physical slowing may resemble parkinsonism

● distinguishing symptoms   cold intolerance

                                         increasing weight

                                         hoarse voice

                                         loss of hair

● distinguishing signs are shown in Figure 17.3

● tests – thyroid function $T_4 \downarrow$

                                   TSH $\uparrow$

investigations

● there are no specific diagnostic tests in idiopathic parkinsonism

● CT scan may be helpful in arteriosclerotic parkinsonism if it is associated with multiple small cerebral infarcts

● nuclear magnetic resonance (NMR) may be helpful in the future since this technique is capable of detecting chemical changes at cellular level, and may be able to demonstrate alteration of dopamine metabolism, which is the basic pathophysiological mechanism underlying parkinsonism

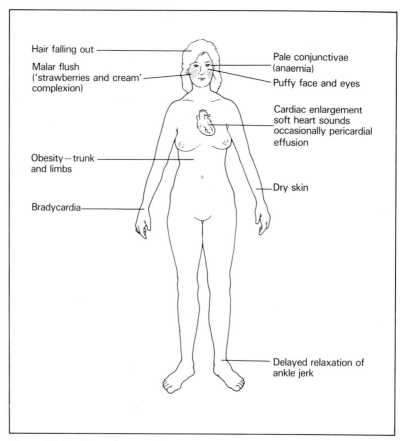

Hair falling out

Malar flush
('strawberries and cream'
complexion)

Pale conjunctivae
(anaemia)

Puffy face and eyes

Cardiac enlargement
soft heart sounds
occasionally pericardial
effusion

Obesity—trunk
and limbs

Dry skin

Bradycardia

Delayed relaxation of
ankle jerk

Figure 17.3   *Signs of myxoedema*

WHAT TO DO?

issues

- no 'cures' are possible
- the only reversible type of parkinsonism is that induced by drugs
- relief with modern medication should be possible in most
- progression may be delayed with drugs
- long course creates great stresses and strains on family who need support and assistance from medical and social services
- many effective drugs now available and should be used selectively in step by step programme

management

general measures

- maintain maximal functional activity through self-help and physiotherapy
- involve local occupational therapist in arrangement for home aids and alterations to prevent accidents and make life easier
- stop any drugs which may be responsible or may aggravate the condition

    phenothiazines (e.g. chlorpromazine)

    tranquillizers

    reserpine

    haloperidol

    methyldopa

medication

- drugs offer best hopes for control of effects of the disease
- step-by-step selective use of drugs

    mild cases – no medication necessary

    tremor – helped by anticholinergics

    rigidity – helped by L-Dopa and other drugs
- the most effective treatment relies on drugs which increase dopaminergic activity

L-Dopa

- replaces dopamine deficiency
- dose

    start 125–500 mg/day

    increase progressively to maximum tolerated dose 2–8 g daily

    make increments slowly

    give divided doses say 4 times/day
- usually combined with decarboxylase inhibitor to allow better blood–brain transmission

- responses

    75% helped + +

    benefits may last 5–10 years but then
    control declines

- side-effects

    nausea and vomiting

    postural hypotension

    tachycardia and other cardiac arrhythmias

    mental changes   agitation

                      hallucinations

                      confusion

                      paranoia

    'on–off' phenomenon – expression of
    duration of effect of the drug – can be
    minimized by dose titration and adjustment
    of the interval between doses

    dyskinesis   grimacing

                      turning/twisting

                      shoulder shrugging

                      tongue jerking

Sinemet

- L-Dopa + dopa-decarboxylase inhibitor
  (Sinemet)

- the inhibitor prevents the peripheral
  breakdown of L-Dopa, thus allowing higher
  concentrations to enter the brain, and also
  reducing the side effects caused by the
  breakdown products of L-Dopa in the circulation

- dose

    start 50 mg 8-hourly

    give dose after meals

    double the dose after 1 week

    slowly increase the dose afterwards to the
    maximum tolerated dose – often 700–800
    mg/day

    always use divided doses – 3–4-hourly best

- *side-effects frequent*
  nausea, vomiting, anorexia
  hypotension, arrhythmias
  involuntary movements
  depression, agitation and aggression

other therapy

- *anticholinergics*
  may be effective in reducing tremor
  drugs
  - benzhexol (Artane) 5–15 mg/day
  - orphenadrine (Disipal) 150–400 mg/day
  - procyclidine (Kemadrin) 7.5–60 mg/day
  special indications
  - tremor +
  - excessive salivation
  - neuroleptic-induced parkinsonism
  side-effects dry mouth
  blurred vision
  urinary retention – especially in elderly with prostate problems
  psychiatric disturbances

- *amantidine*
  moderately effective in improving slowness of movement
  dose 200–400 mg/day
  side-effects nausea/vomiting
  ankle swelling
  confusion

- *bromocriptine*

    dopamine – receptor agonist

    dose 40–140mg/day

    may help to smooth out fluctuations in effectiveness of L-Dopa

    side effects   mental changes

                       dyskinesia

- *selegiline*

    type B monoamine oxidase inhibitor

    potentiates effect of L-Dopa by retarding its breakdown

    dose 10 mg/day

    side-effects   nausea/vomiting

                       dizziness

surgery in Parkinson's disease

- involves destruction of ventrolateral thalamic nucleus through a stereotactic probe under radiographic control
- indicated   younger patient

                   unilateral tremor

                   resistant to drugs

                   otherwise fit and healthy

- tends to be of benefit for limited time only

PROGNOSIS IN PARKINSON'S DISEASE

- average duration of life is 9 years from diagnosis
- mortality rate (observed/expected deaths) is 3 : 1
- 80% of patients severely disabled or dead within 10 years
- 30% of patients ultimately become demented
- most frequent cause of death is bronchopneumonia

Useful practical points

- it is easy to overlook the insidious development of parkinsonism in a patient who is seen frequently for other medical problems
- aching in the shoulders or arms may be an early manifestation of parkinsonism
- a depressed apathetic patient may simulate parkinsonism – it is always worth a trial of antidepressant drugs to see if the condition will improve
- the earliest movement in which to pick up cogwheel rigidity on examination is pronation/supination of the forearm
- senile tremor is most likely to be confused with parkinsonian tremor – the distinguishing feature is that senile tremor is most apparent during active use of the arms, while parkinsonian tremor can improve in these circumstances
- L-Dopa and bromocriptine will help for limited periods only in most patients
- after 10 years of parkinsonism most patients are depressed, demented and housebound

18

RHEUMATOID ARTHRITIS

WHAT IS IT?

- a multisystem disease
- joints are target organs
- basic pathology is inflammation with tissue damage, destruction and repair (to limited extent)
- systemic changes are variable
- different presentations, patterns and degrees of disability (almost different diseases)

diagnostic criteria (American Rheumatism Association)

- morning stiffness
- pain on movement or tenderness in at least one joint
- swelling in at least two joints
- symmetrical joint swelling – same joint both sides
- subcutaneous nodules
- presence of rheumatoid factor
- poor mucin precipitate from synovial fluid
- characteristic histology in synovial membrane
- characteristic histology in nodules

classification according to ARA

- definite RA – five of above criteria for at least 6 weeks
- classic RA – seven criteria for 6 weeks
- probable RA – three criteria for at least 4 weeks

aetiology	• cause is unknown
	• auto-immune disorder
	either failure of suppressor T cells or stimulation of B cells
	proliferation of lymphocytes and plasma cells in joint capsule lining and elsewhere
	hypergammaglobulinaemia
	rheumatoid factor production (80% of cases) – present in blood and joint fluid
	• trigger unknown – possibly a virus
	• genetic predisposition – tissue type HLA-DR4 is particularly prone to develop the disease (HLA–DR3 has more severe disease)
	• environmental factors – higher incidence in urbanized Africans than those in primitive communities
WHO GETS IT AND WHEN?	• worldwide distribution
	• probably an ancient disease
	• no good evidence of any increase or decrease in prevalence
	• F > M by 3 : 1
prevalence	• 1–2% of population has 'active' disease
	• probably up to 4% of population has rheumatoid arthritis at some time (in many it remits or is quiescent)
age of onset	• peak at 20–40 years
	• can occur at any age

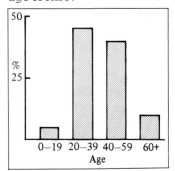

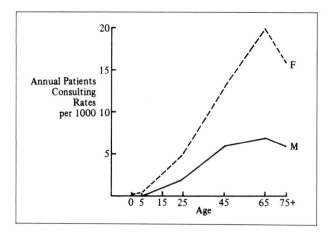

age prevalence

- most prevalent in middle age
- F > M but less so in elderly

frequency

general practice

general practice with 2500 persons: rheumatoid arthritis

Annual new cases (incidence)	2

Annual patients consulting (prevalence)	25
(severe	6)
(very severe	2)

district general hospital

DGH 250 000 population: rheumatoid arthritis

Annual admissions	100

Annual persons attending OPD	1000

(Very severely disabled in population	200)

history

onset

- abrupt in 20% with rapidly developing polyarthritis and severe constitutional symptoms (may be monarticular)
- most develop over weeks or months

symptoms

- *general* malaise

  increased fatigue

  poor appetite

  weight loss

  low grade fever; sweats

- *joints*

  pain and swelling of multiple joints with loss
  of movement and function

  frequency of involvement (Figure 18.1)

  most   proximal interphalangeal

  metacarpophalangeal

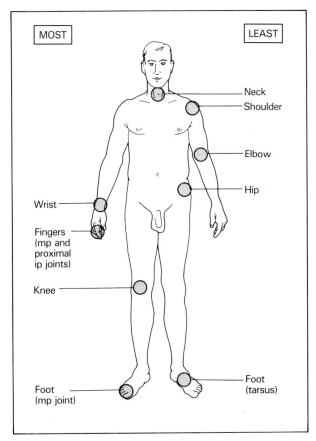

Figure 18.1   *Joint involvement in RA*

wrists

metatarsophalangeal

knees

least elbows

shoulders

tarsus

ankles

hips

neck

pain present at rest but worse on activity

affected joints stiff especially after inactivity most marked early morning – lasts more than 30 minutes

a distinctive feature is symmetrical involvement of the joints

- *other symptoms due to systemic involvement*

  painful eyes – scleritis, episcleritis

  pleuritic pain/pericarditic pain

  cold white fingers – Raynaud's phenomenon

  breathlessness – pulmonary involvement

  paraesthesiae – polyneuropathy

  painful muscles – myositis

  diarrhoea – amyloid

  symptoms of anaemia

- the extent of joint involvement correlates poorly with extra-articular manifestations

- *family history* – there may be a family history of rheumatoid arthritis or other immune disorders

  pernicious anaemia

  myxoedema (Hashimoto's thyroiditis)

  ulcerative colitis (Crohn's disease)

  hypoparathyroidism

  diabetes

examination : joints

- acute disease
  - hot red joint
  - fusiform (spindle-shaped) swelling
  - limited movement
  - symmetrical involvement
  - fine crepitus
- chronic disease
  - swollen deformed joints
  - ulnar deviation hand
  - 'swan-neck' deformity of fingers (Figure 18.2)
  - flexion deformity or valgus/varus deformity of the knees
  - immobility of the wrist
  - flexion contracture of elbow
  - coarse crepitus in joints if associated with osteoarthritis

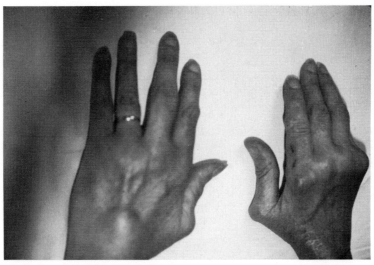

Figure 18.2   *Photograph of deformities in hands due to rheumatoid arthritis*

possible findings are shown in Figure 18.3

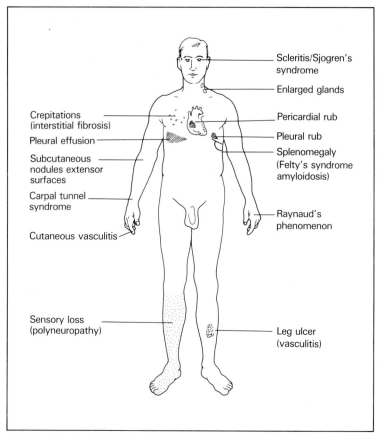

Figure 18.3 *Possible extra-articular findings on examination in rheumatoid arthritis*

investigations

blood tests

- for anaemia

  normochromic normocytic – usual type

  iron deficiency – due to chronic blood loss from drug treatment

  rare

  mild haemolysis

  macrocytic (due to low serum folate)

RHEUMATOID ARTHRITIS

- for pancytopenia
    - Felty's syndrome
    - drug-induced
- for evidence of activity
    - ESR
    - white cell count
    - plasma viscosity (1.5 – 1.7 cP)
    - C-reactive protein (0–20 μg/ml)
    - hyperfibrinogenaemia (2–4g/l)
- immunology
    - rheumatoid factor 80%
    - antinuclear antibodies 30%
    - DNA – binding test 20%
    - if vasculitis present
        - circulating immune complexes
        - cryoglobulins
        - low level of complement
- alkaline phosphatase may be increased in active disease

radiology

joints

the X-ray changes of rheumatoid arthritis are best seen in the hands

- juxta-articular osteoporosis
- narrow joint space due to loss of cartilage
- marginal and cystic erosions
    - metacarpal heads
    - proximal phalangeal heads
    - carpal bones
    - head of radius and ulna

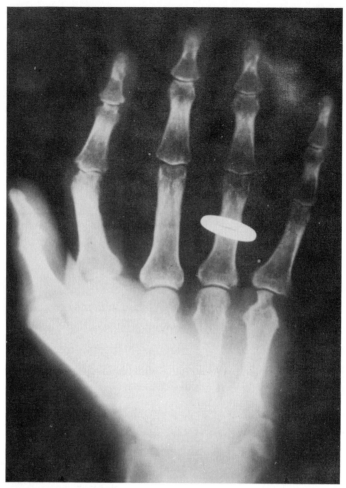

Figure 18.4 *X-ray hand in rheumatoid arthritis showing juxta-articular osteoporosis and also cystic erosions round the metacarpo-phalangeal joint of the index finger*

- dislocations and joint deformities

  a typical X-ray of the hands in rheumatoid arthritis is shown in Figure 18.4

chest X-ray

- pleural effusion 20%
- rheumatoid nodules alone
- rheumatoid nodules + massive fibrosis in coalminers (Caplan's syndrome)
- interstitial fibrosis

RHEUMATOID ARTHRITIS

analysis of synovial fluid	• cloudy yellow
	• low viscosity
	• increased protein
	• clots easily
	• WBC, 2000 – 75 000/mm (polymorphs > 50%)
	• complement low – important finding

special types of rheumatoid arthritis

juvenile (Still's disease)	three types
	• systemic
	• polyarthritic
	• pauci-articular (< 5 joints)

systemic	• 1–5 years
	• high remittent temperature
	• maculopapular/erythematous rash
	• lymphadenopathy
	• splenomegaly
	• arthralgia knees
	wrists
	carpi
	ankles
	tarsi

polyarthritic	• girls > boys
	• any age
	• acute or insidious onset
	• extensive polyarthritis small joints
	• neck often involved
	• tenosynovitis common
	• growth retardation

pauci-articular	• commonest – two out of three cases
	• knees, ankles, elbows most frequent
	• tenosynovitis often
	• may persist in single joint for years
	• iridocyclitis common
	• usually 1–5 years old, equal sex incidence

elderly

- may begin > 65 years old: sexes equal
- three presentations

    insidious in a few joints

    acute polyarthritis

    limb girdle involvement like polymyalgia rheumatica

- milder with less deformity than in young
- anaemia common
- extra-articular manifestations uncommon
- drug treatment more likely to be associated with side-effects

differential diagnosis of rheumatoid arthritis

systemic lupus erythematosus (SLE)

- the features are shown in Figure 18.5
- the differentiation between rheumatoid arthritis and SLE is as follows

RA	SLE
Middle-aged woman	Young woman
Gradual onset	Acute onset
± Constitutional symptoms	Severe constitutional upset
Small joints – symmetrical	Small joints – asymmetrical
Constant pain	Flitting joint pain
Deformity very common	Deformity very rare
Morning stiffness common	No morning stiffness
No rash	Typical butterfly rash
Other systems infrequent	Other systems often
X-ray – destructive lesions	Bony lesions rare

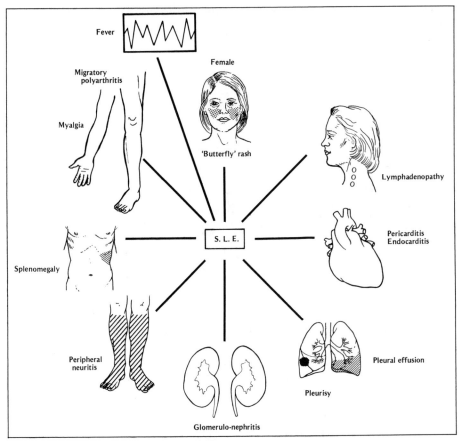

Figure 18.5 *Features of SLE*

- tests

    antinuclear antibodies test (99% cases of SLE)

    DNA binding test – virtually invariable in SLE (has replaced LE test)

    antilymphocytic antibodies – common in SLE – rare in RA

polymyalgia rheumatica

- the features are shown in Figure 18.6
- distinctive points   usually males

onset > 60

larger joints affected

hips

shoulders

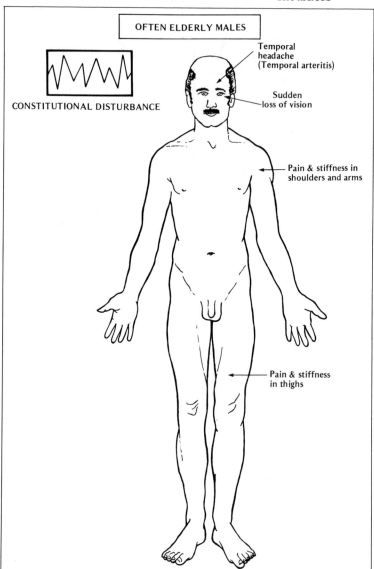

Figure 18.6   *Features of polymyalgia rheumatica*

- tests   very high ESR

        rheumatoid factor negative

rheumatic fever

- young age groups
- migratory joint pains
- evidence of rheumatic carditis

    systolic murmur

    diastolic murmur (Carey–Coombs)

    cardiac enlargement

- subcutaneous nodules common
- erythema marginatum often
- choreiform movements occasionally present
- tests

    increase in antistreptolysin titre

    e.c.g. evidence of myocarditis

    echocardiographic evidence of rheumatic vegetations on the mitral valve

gouty arthritis

- usually only one joint involved

    1st metatarsophalangeal commonest

    also foot, ankle, knee

- 90% males (unlike RA – predominance of females)
- attacks often at night
- tophi in ears, elbows or hands in chronic gout
- tests

    raised serum uric acid

    X-ray – distinctive peripheral articular cartilage erosions and bone cysts (Figure 18.7)

    synovial fluid – urate crystals

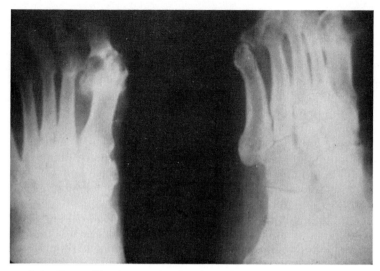

Figure 18.7 *X-ray of feet in gout showing gross disorganization and erosion of first metatarso-phalangeal joints*

infective (septic) arthritis

- red, hot, shiny, swollen joint
- usually monarticular
- may be an infective focus elsewhere
- may be associated with steroid treatment of rheumatoid arthritis
- severe constitutional symptoms
- tests

    high white cell (polymorphonuclear) count

    changes in synovial fluid

      turbid green

      high white cell count ($> 100\,000/\text{mm}^3$)

      organisms on film/culture

psoriatic arthritis

- terminal interphalangeal joints involved
- nail beds often pitted and ridged
- long history of psoriasis with psoriatic patches on skin
- ankylosing spondylitis may be present
- tests – rheumatoid factor negative

osteoarthrosis	• degenerative disease later in life
	• major joint usually affected, especially weight-bearing
	• if hands affected → terminal interphalangeal joints
	• joints rarely affected symmetrically
	• no systemic disturbances
	• tests

ESR normal

rheumatoid factor absent

X-ray

osteophytes

articular osteosclerosis

WHAT HAPPENS? a simple functional grading is helpful in assessing disability

in the home	getting in/out of bed
	washing/bathing
	dressing
	walking up/down stairs
	housework
outside	getting about
	shopping
	working

• grading

1 completely independent home/work
2 independent with aids/appliances
3 partially dependent – help necessary in dressing and toilet function
4 completely dependent – confined to bed or wheelchair

outcomes

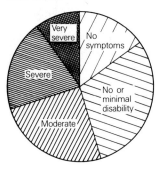

- no symptoms
- no or minimal disability } (grade 1 above)
- moderate disability (grade 2)
- severe disability (grade 3)
- very severe disability – cannot live independently (grade 4)

Grades	1	2	3	4	
%	45	25	20	10	100

course

possible courses

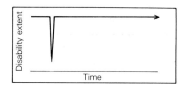

single episode of mono/polyarthritis with full recovery and no recurrence

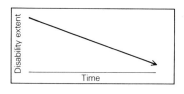

slow steady progressive disease

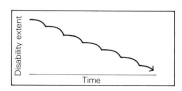

progressive deterioration with acute episodes

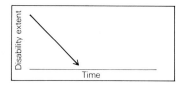

rapid deterioration with severe disability

RHEUMATOID ARTHRITIS

issues

- rheumatoid arthritis is a chronic disabling demoralizing disease which is a burden on the patient, on the relatives and on the doctor

- the cause is unknown and no effective 'cures' are available

- the disease often follows a steady deteriorating course with significant effects on the general health and independence of the patient, and may shorten life if severe vasculitis or other extra-articular complications are present

- the doctor's job is to ensure that the patient will be able to live with the disease based on a multidisciplinary approach involving drugs to relieve symptoms, physiotherapy, occupational therapy, social services help and psychological support for the patient and his family

- the aims of treatment therefore are to relieve pain, to make the best of what function is available, to attain as much independence as possible and to improve and maintain morale

MANAGEMENT OF RHEUMATOID ARTHRITIS

most patients with chronic rheumatoid arthritis can be successfully managed at home by GP

indications for hospital referral

- GP may want help with treatment

- patient/family dissatisfied with lack of progress

- special problems

    surgery to be considered

    septic arthritis

    atypical picture ? underlying collagen disorder

- severe acute exacerbations – often settles better initially in hospital than at home

acute phase treatment

general measures

- bed rest till symptoms/signs disappear
- firm mattress or bedboards
- minimum pillows
- foot cage
- regular thigh/foot exercise to prevent venous thrombosis
- high calorie diet/ample protein

local measures

- immobilization acutely painful joints in good functional position by plaster-of-Paris splints
- remove splints for active non-weightbearing exercises when pain and swelling subsides
- heat to relieve stiffness/pain
- wax baths for stiffness hands/feet
- exercises to maintain muscles around joint as soon as acute phase subsided

drugs

- *aspirin* in first choice in maximum tolerated dose – 4–6 g daily

    side-effects   dizziness

    tinnitus/impaired hearing

    GI upsets

    indigestion

    bleeding

- *non-steroidal anti-inflammatory drugs (NSAI)*

    effective second line treatment

    many preparations available – best to become thoroughly familiar with potential and side-effects of a few

    naproxen 250–500 mg b.d.

    indomethacin (Indocid) 25–50 mg 2 or 3 times daily

    ibuprofen (Brufen) 200 mg – 400 mg 2–3 times daily

    piroxicam (Feldene) 10–30 mg daily

usage

    one drug at a time

    prescribe adequate dose

    prescribe for limited time

side-effects

    gastric irritation – least likely with fenbufen and ibuprofen

    gastrointestinal bleeding

    fluid retentions   oedema

                      hypertension

    hypersensitivity   angioneurotic oedema

                      asthma

                      trashes

    headache

    vertigo and tinnitus

    blood dyscrasias – rare

drug interaction with NSAI drugs

    anticoagulants, e.g. warfarin

    antidiabetics, e.g. tolbutamide

    diuretics

    antihypertensive drugs

    anticonvulsants, e.g. phenytoin

long term treatment

general

- education

    nature of the disease

    prognosis

    benefits as well as limitation of available treatment

- support – assurance of continuous support from GP

- iron – if iron-deficiency anaemia due to chronic GI blood loss from treatment

	• treatment of depression
	encouragement
	antidepressive drugs

physiotherapy
- exercises to improve and maintain muscle and joint function
- strengthen quadriceps after periods of prolonged bed rest
- avoid joint trauma from inappropriate and stressful use
- hydrotherapy to improve muscle function without weight-bearing
- heat   to relieve pain

    to relieve spasm
- ice to reduce joint swelling
- swimming is excellent exercise

occupational therapy
- splinting to preserve hand function
- assess all activities including hobbies and advise on how best to carry out
- appliances and gadgets to continue household tasks
- special fixtures and fittings in kitchen and bathroom

drugs
- NSAIs as necessary
- 'slow-acting' drugs if inadequate control with other treatment

antimalarials
- chloroquine 250 mg a day hydroxychloroquine 200 mg b.d.
- improvement in 50% in 4–12 weeks
- main side-effect is retinal damage – should have ophthalmic check every 6 months

	● other side-effects	nausea
		diarrhoea
		rashes
		dizziness/deafness
		haemolytic anaemia

penicillamine

● indications

  active progressive disease in spite of other treatment

  nodules + high titre of rheumatoid factor

  extra-articular disease

● dose – 125–250 mg orally to start, increase by up to 250 mg monthly to maximum 1 g/day

● improvement 50–60%

● side-effects   rashes

         loss of taste

         vomiting

         fever

         mouth ulcers

         proteinuria/nephrotic syndrome

         pancytopenia

gold (chrysotherapy)

● indications – as for penicillamine

● dose – test dose 10 mg
         i.m. 50 mg weekly till response (2–3 months) then continued less frequently for as long as required

● side-effects   rashes

         mouth ulcers

         enterocolitis

         nephrotic syndrome

         pancytopenia

steroid treatment

- indications

    very severe exacerbations, unresponsive to rest and NSAI

    to control persistently disabling disease in young mothers or breadwinners when other measures have failed

    severe extra-articular disease, e.g. scleritis, vasculitis

- prednisolone is best drug – use smallest dose necessary to control the disease and preferably no more than 7.5 mg/day to avoid adrenal suppression

- side-effects   Cushingoid appearance

    fluid retention

        moon-face

        oedema

        hypertension

    peptic ulcer

    diabetes

    spontaneous bruising

    osteoporosis – fractures

    psychosis

    susceptibility to infection

- local intra-articular injections of hydrocortisone are also useful in acute exacerbations

immunotherapy

- indications

    life-threatening extra-articular manifestations unresponsive to all other treatment

    severe progressive unresponsive disease

    to allow lower dose of steroids

- drugs

    azathioprine 1.25–2.5 mg/kg

    cyclophosphamide 1–2 mg/kg

- side-effects alopecia

　　　　　　　　nausea/vomiting

　　　　　　　　bone marrow suppression

　　　　　　　　susceptibility to infection

　　　　　　　　carcinogenic potential

social services　　these may be very helpful in the chronically disabled housebound patient

home nurses
- bathing/washing help
- check and advise on medication to be taken
- assess and arrange provision of aids, e.g. walking sticks, commode etc
- encourage and support

social worker
- counselling on finance with limited budget
- advice on welfare rights

　　　attendance allowance

　　　mobility allowance

　　　heating allowance
- provision of home help
- arrange meals-on-wheels/luncheon club
- arrange attendance at day centre if possible
- arrange night-sitters if required
- assess housing requirements

SURGERY IN RHEUMATOID ARTHRITIS

indications

- severe unremitting pain unresponsive to medical treatment
- severe loss of necessary joint function
- severe instability of a joint
- unacceptable loss of joint mobility

- progressive joint destruction on X-ray

types of surgery available

- synovectomy
- reconstructive tendon surgery
- arthroplasty
- arthrodesis

ALTERNATIVE TREATMENT – ACUPUNCTURE

- acupuncture is being used increasingly in musculoskeletal disorders including rheumatoid arthritis
- claimed to relieve

  pain

  stiffness

  swelling of joints and muscles

- has no effect on bony abnormalities
- six to ten treatments required
- relief of pain may last from 6 months to 5 years
- treatment involves mechanical or electrical stimulation of a needle placed in certain 'meridian' points remote from the painful site. The analgesic effect might be due to release of endogenous analgesic substances (endorphins): the effects can be reversed by the use of the morphine antagonist, naloxone
- more controlled clinical trials with objective assessment of progress are required before the place of acupuncture in chronic rheumatoid arthritis can be satisfactorily evaluated

Useful practical points
- rheumatoid arthritis is a general systemic disorder and not just a disease of the joints
- it is important to educate both the patient and his relatives in the natural history of the disease and the benefits and limitations of treatment
- aspirin is probably the best drug for initial treatment of an acute exacerbation but be alert to the possibility of side-effects, especially in the elderly
- hypochromic anaemia is common in longstanding rheumatoid arthritis due to gastrointestinal blood loss caused by treatment
- most of the non-steroidal anti-inflammatory drugs have similar efficacy though side-effects may differ slightly: become thoroughly familiar with only a few but use them in optimal dosage
- steroids should only be used long term when all other methods have failed, and then in the lower possible dose, preferably not over 7.5 mg/day
- depression is frequent in chronic disease and may require effective antidepressant drugs, but use these for the minimum time possible

19   LOW BACKACHE

WHAT IS IT?

- backache is the consequence of the human two-legged stance
- with over 50 bones, 100 joints and 1000 muscles and ligaments transmitting most of the body weight, it is scarcely surprising that this complex structure is prone to complex disorders
- almost everyone suffers from backache at some time of their lives, most is minor, transient and self-resolving
- there is poor correlation between the pathology and the clinical pictures – probably because, since backache is a benign non-killing condition, there are few possibilities of demonstrating the morbid anatomy and pathology
- therefore the clinician has to rely on appreciation of symptoms, signs and likely course and outcome to manage patients with backache
- it is useful to divide low backache into 'acute' and 'chronic' varieties, although the two may merge into each other
- the *acute back* is of sudden onset and relatively short duration, the *chronic back* goes on and on

causes of low backache

mechanical

- prolapsed intervertebral disc
- osteoarthrosis (osteoarthritis)
- injuries/fractures

- spinal stenosis
- congenital   spondylolisthesis
           spina bifida
           transitional vertebrae
- juvenile osteochondritis (Scheuermann's disease)
- functional strain – occupational etc

inflammatory

- ankylosing spondylitis
- tuberculosis of the spine
- rheumatoid arthritis
- osteomyelitis

metabolic

- osteoporosis
     spontaneous in elderly
     iatrogenic – steroid treatment
- osteomalacia
- hyperparathyroidism

neoplastic

- bone
     metastases – commonest
     myeloma
     reticulosis, e.g. Hodgkin's disease
     primary – osteosarcoma
- spinal tumours, e.g. meningioma, glioma

referred pain

- abdomen
     aorta   dissection
           aneurysm
     peptic ulcer
     gallbladder disease
     pancreatic disease

- pelvis
    salpingitis
    cervicitis
    prolapsed uterus – rare
    endometriosis

Paget's disease

psychogenic

- anxiety/depression
- compensation
- malingering

WHO GETS IT WHEN?

acute

acute backache is a condition of active adults, equally affecting men and women

chronic

chronic backache is prevalent from 40 onwards, but can affect younger adults also

risk factors

- heavy physical work
- poor static posture
- bending, lifting, twisting
- car driving (truck drivers have fewer backaches than car and tractor drivers)

age prevalence

- *children*   Scheuermann's disease
              congenital disorders

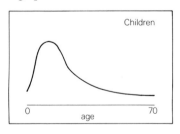

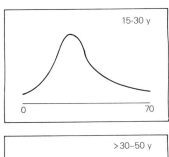

- *15–30 years* prolapsed disc
  traumatic fractures
  ankylosing spondylitis
  spondylolisthesis

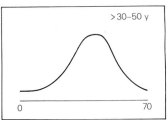

- *> 30–50 years* chronic prolapsed disc
  malignancy
  dissecting aneurysm
  functional strain

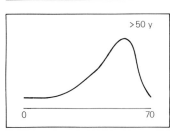

- *> 50 years* osteoarthrosis
  Paget's disease
  malignancy
  atheromatous abdominal
  aneurysm
  senile osteoporosis
  spinal stenosis

frequency

general practice

low backache in a practice population of 2500

Acute back	
Annual *incidence* of new cases	75
Chronic back	
Annual *prevalence* of patients consulting	50
(*Back invalids*	3–4)

district general hospital

DGH serving 250 000 population (estimated):
low backache – annual numbers

Referred to outpatient department	
Acute	400
Chronic	500
Admitted	
Acute	30
Chronic	40

WHAT HAPPENS?

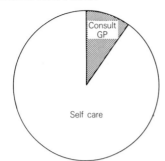

- it is estimated that only one in ten of those with backache consults their GP

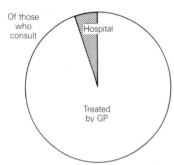

- of those seen by *GP*, 5% are referred to hospital but more than half of these recover before being seen and do not attend OP

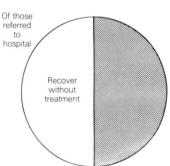

- of those treated at *hospital* one half recover during investigations and before any treatment is given

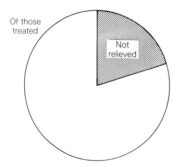

- of those *actually treated at hospital*, 20% are *not* relieved and have persistent symptoms
- of all backache patients seen by the GP, one in 1000 eventually has *surgery*
- of those *treated surgically*, over 10% continue to suffer chronic backache

- *rates of surgery* are different in various countries

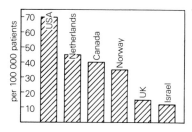

Laminectomy per 100 000 population	
USA	70
(Western 90)	
Netherlands	45
Canada	40
Norway	35
UK	15
Israel	12

acute back

clinical types

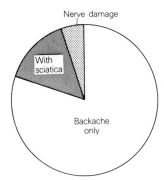

- *presentation of acute back – general practice*

    acute backache only – 80%

    acute backache with sciatica – 15%

    acute backache with nerve damage – 5%

WHAT HAPPENS?

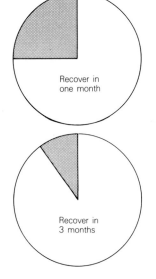

- 75% of all acute backs recover (with minimal treatment) in 1 month

- 90% of all acute backs recover in 3 months
- each GP with 2500 patients will have three to four disabled back invalids in spite of multiple forms of treatments

WHAT TO DO?

issues

- backache is very common but should not be treated with contempt: it may be crippling and it may be caused by serious disease
- the proven cause of most backaches is uncertain and the nature of the disorder likewise is unclear
- understanding and management have to be pragmatic
- since majority of backaches tend to resolve spontaneously, it is difficult to assess the value of treatments
- there are many treatments available and many professionals and paraprofessionals willing to treat
- essentially the major issues are: which patients should be treated with more than simple methods and who should do the treating?

diagnosis

history

onset

   acute

- acute prolapsed intervertebral disc
- compression fracture

     osteoporosis

     neoplasia

- acute osteomyelitis
- traumatic fracture
- acute referred pain

     dissecting aneurysm

     peptic ulcer

     acute cholecystitis

     acute pancreatitis

chronic	• lumbago/sciatica syndrome
	chronic prolapsed disc
	osteoarthrosis
	• ankylosing spondylitis
	• tuberculosis of the spine
	• congenital
	spondylolisthesis
	transitional vertebra
	• Paget's disease
	• chronic functional back strain
	• psychogenic

character	• most are dull aching pain
	• burning pain (often down the leg) → nerve root compression
	• acute localized excruciating pain → spontaneous fracture of vertebra
	• dull throbbing pain → abdominal aneurysm with vertebral erosion
	• progressively more severe → malignancy
	• diffuse pain → systemic inflammatory disease, e.g. ankylosing spondylitis
	• cramping pain → muscle spasm

radiation	• into leg and foot → prolapsed disc
	• into buttock and thigh → spinal stenosis
	• anterior aspects thighs/legs → lesion in upper lumbar vertebrae
	• gluteal region, posterior thigh/calf → lesion in lower lumbar/sacral vertebrae
	• from abdomen into back → visceral disease
	peptic ulcer
	gallbladder disease
	pancreatic disease

aggravation	• movement → mechanical back pain (see pages 318–319)
	• coughing/sneezing/straining/lifting → mechanical pain, especially prolapsed disc lesion
	• walking → spinal stenosis
	• at night in bed →
	malignancy
	inflammatory disease
relief	• rest/immobility → mechanical pain especially PID
	• sitting and flexing spine →
	spinal stenosis
	pancreatitis
past history	• operation for malignancy, e.g. cancer of breast → back pain due to metastasis (even after many years)
	• psychiatric illness → 'psychogenic' backache
family history	• neurofibromatosis → pain from root irritation by neurofibroma
	• rheumatoid arthritis/ankylosing spondylitis
	• inflammatory bowel disease (ulcerative colitis/ Crohn's disease) → ankylosing spondylitis
examination	• *general* findings which may be relevant are shown in Figure 19.1
	• *examination of the spine*
	appearance
	scoliosis → disc lesion
	flattening of lumbosacral spine →
	disc lesion
	inflammatory disease

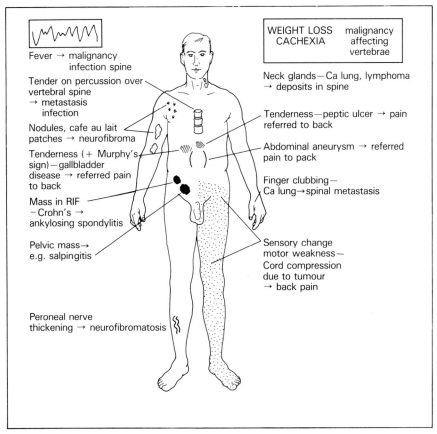

Figure 19.1   *Possible general findings in back pain*

localized angulation (gibbus) →
vertebral collapse

metastasis

osteoporosis

flexion at the hip/knee → disc prolapse

dorsal kyphosis, rigid spine → ankylosing
spondylitis

mobility

limited forward flexion →

degenerative disease

disc lesion

limited lateral flexion one side only →

  disc lesion

  degenerative disease

lateral flexion limited both sides →

  ankylosing spondylitis

tenderness on percussion →

  infection

  neoplasia

- *straight-leg raising* < 90% → sciatic nerve irritation

  disc lesion

  osteoarthrosis

- *femoral stretch test* (flex knee then extend hip) – pain in anterior part of thigh indicates femoral root irritation

- *sacroiliac joint*

  press over dimples in low lumbar area

  press over sacrum with patient prone

  pain in either test → ankylosing spondylitis

- *neurological examination*

  muscle weakness, depressed reflexes and sensory change indicates serious organic disease

  the changes which occur with prolapsed lumbosacral discs are shown in Figure 19.2

  spinal cord compression (tumours)

    upper lumbar

      normal motor function

      extensor plantars

      bowel/bladder dysfunction

    cauda equina

      lower motor neuron type of leg weakness

      normal plantars

      bowel/bladder dysfunction

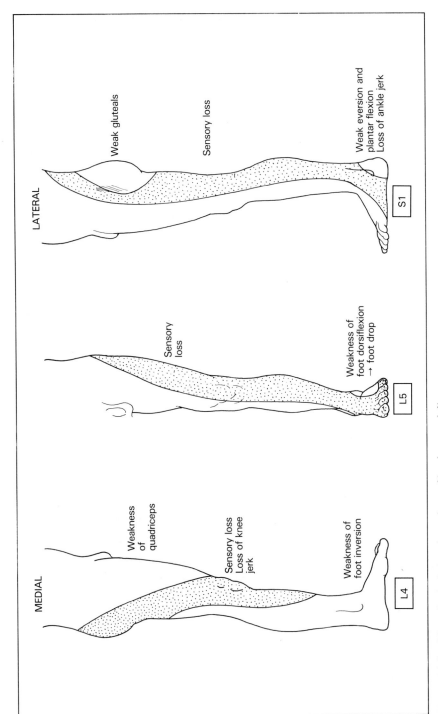

Figure 19.2 *Neurological signs in prolapsed lumbosacral discs*

inflammatory disease

    wasting of paraspinal muscles

    multiple root involvement

    other neurological signs originating from spinal cord involvement

investigations

- *not necessary in most patients*
- *indications*   root compression

                  spinal cord compression

                  suspected disease of vertebrae

                  surgical treatment considered

radiology

- plain X-ray spine

    osteophytes → osteoarthrosis (Figure 19.3)

    narrow disc space → PID

    vertebral destruction → tumour (Figure 19.4)

                                    infection

    congenital abnormalities   spondylolisthesis

                                    transitional vertebra

                                    spina bifida

    osteoporosis ± vertebral collapse → senile osteoporosis

    sclerosis → metastases cancer prostate (Figure 19.5)

                          Paget's disease

    sacroiliitis → ankylosing spondylitis (Figure 19.6)

    'bamboo spine' → ankylosing spondylitis

- tomography – more sensitive in detecting bone destruction

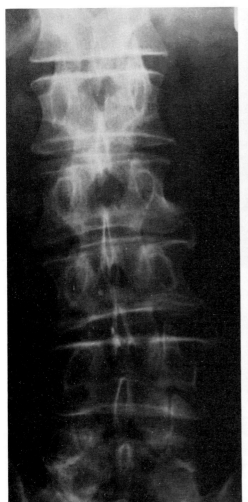

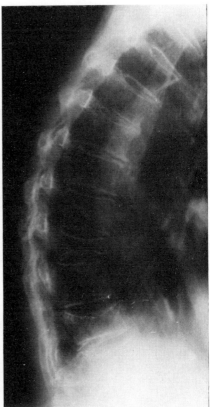

Figure 19.4 *X-ray spine showing a collapsed vertebra due to myeloma*

Figure 19.3 *X-ray of the spine in osteo-arthrosis showing marked osteophyte formation (lipping) and narrowed disc spaces*

- myelography – detection of compressive lesions

  discs

  tumours

  abscess

- radiculography – has largely replaced myelography in disc lesions

- discography – helpful in multiple disc lesions

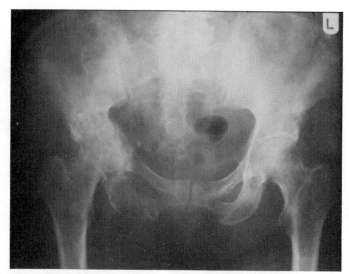

Figure 19.5 *X-ray spine and pelvis showing osteosclerotic and osteoclastic metastases due to carcinoma of the prostate*

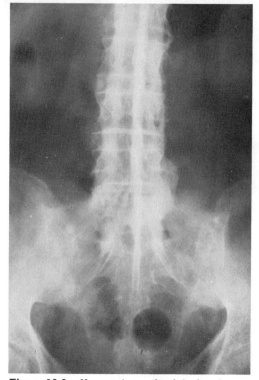

Figure 19.6 *X-ray spine and pelvis showing 'bamboo' spine due to ankylosing spondylitis*

- CT scan can detect

  eroded vertebral bodies

  herniated discs

  spinal cord tumours

  tumours in intervertebral foramina, e.g. neurofibroma

  paravertebral masses

- epidural venography – for laterally-herniated discs

- spinal angiography for

  tumour of spinal cord

  vascular malformations in spinal cord

blood tests

- ESR – increased in

  inflammatory disease

  neoplastic disease

- calcium level

  increased   carcinomatosis

                 myelomatosis

  lowered   osteomalacia

- phosphate level   lowered in osteomalacia

- phosphatase level

  alkaline

     increased   malignancy

                    osteomalacia

                    Paget's disease (++)

  acid – increased in cancer prostate especially with metastases

lumbar puncture

- c.s.f. may show malignant cells

- pathogenic organisms in c.s.f.

isotope bone scan

- for detecting bone tumours – primary and secondary

TREATMENT

issues

- since most backaches are benign and resolve spontaneously, do not rush into unnecessary active therapy
- since most backaches are caused by mechanical functional stresses and strains, *rest* should be a first step
- take care not to miss major disease as a cause
- *relief of pain* by analgesics and other drugs
- *physical measures* should be undertaken for specific indications and with definite objectives
- *surgery* is a physical treatment to which above provisos apply

management of low back pain

general measures

- explain nature (as far as is known) and likely cause
- consider prevention for future
    avoid bending spine
    correct lifting procedure
    control weight
    appropriate chairs and beds
    correct work-surface height
- advise on rest
- arrange follow-up

specific treatment for mechanical back pain

- complete bed rest – firm mattress
- analgesics
    oral   mild – paracetamol
        strong
            dihydrocodeine (DF118)
            buprenorphine (Temgesic)
            Diconal

intramuscular   pentazocine (Fortral)

                           buprenorphine

                           dihydrocodeine

- an additional tranquillizer may help, e.g.

  diazepam

  nitrazepam (night)

- indications for traction

  persisting pain

  progressive neurological symptoms or signs

- manipulation may help in giving quicker relief from pain but should be restricted to patients without neurological involvement

- exercises are started when the pain has subsided after the period of immobilization

- indications for lumbar support

  patient needs to remain ambulant

  heat/traction ineffective in producing long term benefit

  no relief with bed rest

  manipulation contraindicated

- epidural injection local anaesthetic/steroid – effective in severe unremitting sciatica

- chemonucleolysis – direct injection of chymopapain into affected disc nucleus – effective in relieving pain in 80% of patients with acute disc lesions

- indications for surgery

  persistence of severe pain in spite of full medical treatment

  progressive neurological signs especially lesions of cauda equina causing bladder/ bowel symptoms

  unacceptable recurrence rate of the disc lesion

Useful practical points

- chronic back pain without evidence of an organic cause may be a manifestation of discontent with work and lack of job satisfaction

- the majority of patients with disc prolapse require no tests and will settle quite satisfactorily with bed rest alone

- sudden onset of acute mid-dorsal back pain in a middle-aged patient with no previous back problems is highly likely to be due to a vertebral metastasis; in an elderly patient the most likely cause is vertebral collapse associated with senile osteoporosis

- remember the possibility of osteoporosis and pathological fracture in patients on long term steroids for rheumatoid arthritis or asthma

- many disc problems will recur – 'once a bad back always a bad back'

- lack of bladder control in a patient with back pain is an urgent indication for surgical exploration of the cauda equina

20   URINARY TRACT INFECTIONS

WHAT IS IT?

Medical Research Council Bacteriuria Committee definitions:

- urinary tract infection (UTI) is the presence of micro-organisms in the urinary tract (Figure 20.1)

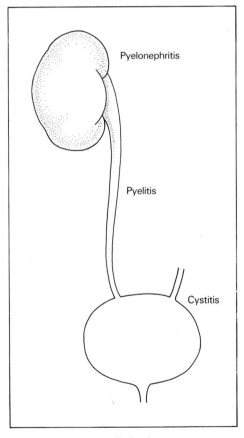

Figure 20.1   *Sites of infection*

- *bacteriuria* denotes the presence of bacteria in bladder urine. It is significant if there are more than 10^8 colony forming units per litre of freshly voided urine ($>$ 100 000 organisms/ml urine)

    bladder bacteriuria may be detected either from midstream specimen, or catheter or suprapubic aspiration

    covert (asymptomatic) bacteriuria denotes significant bacteriuria detected in screening of apparently healthy populations

    frequency and dysuria syndrome ('cystitis') may be bacterial or abacterial

    bacterial cystitis – day and night frequency and dysuria with bacteriuria and pyuria and often haematuria (50% all cases)

    abacterial cystitis (urethral syndrome) frequency and dysuria but no bladder bacteria detected (49%)

    acute bacterial pyelonephritis with loin pains, fever and bacteriuria, bacteraemia, pyuria and haematuria (1%)

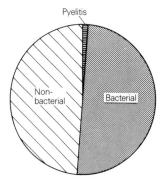

causes

- the exact aetiology and pathogenesis of UTI are speculative and confusing because of difficulties in relating common symptoms (dysuria and frequency) to gross pathological abnormalities

- distinction has to be made between *symptoms* of UTI (dysuria and frequency) and *signs* of UTI, i.e. bacteriuria

- features of UTI may be *functional* and occur in apparently normal intact urinary tracts and *structural* when associated with diseased urinary tracts

functional

- _functional (with normal urinary tract)_

    most often in women with symptoms
    (dysuria and frequency)

    possibly because of impaired defence
    mechanisms

    Impairment of defence mechanisms

    increasing age
    vesico-ureteral reflux
    obstructive uropathy, e.g. stones
    hypertension → renal damage
    chronic prostatitis in men

    possible factors   sexual intercourse

                                    cold weather

                                    emotional upsets

                                    allergies (food and
                                    drinks)

                                    pregnancy

                                    catheterization

structural

- _structural (with possible diseased urinary
    tract)_: different causes in at-risk groups

    children

    congenital abnormalities (rare)

    urethral obstructions (valves and
    strictures)

    hydronephrosis

    vesico-ureteric reflux

    phimosis (rare)

    men

    bladder neck obstruction – prostatic

    urethral strictures

    calculi – bladder/kidney

    kidney disorders – hydronephrosis

women

> urethral stricture (often post-traumatic after pregnancy)
>
> prolapse – cystocoele
>
> calculi – bladder/kidney
>
> kidney disorders – hydronephrosis

elderly

> bladder neck obstructions
>
> atonic bladder

pathogens

% of cases in which bacteria isolated in UTI

	General practice	Hospitals
Escherichia coli	73	41
Staphylococcus albus	6	6.5
Proteus mirabilis	5.7	10.8
Klebsiella	4.8	13.6
Streptococcus fecalis	3.4	12.1
Pseudomonas pyocyanea	1.4	4.8

WHO GETS IT WHEN?

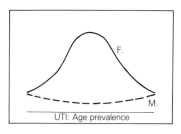

UTI: Age prevalence

- UTI are more prevalent in females than males at all ages (F : M = 5:1) : up to 30% of all women have symptoms of urinary tract infection some time in their lives

- in males prevalence is highest in infancy and old age

- *annual incidence* (new cases) is seven per 1000

- *annual prevalence* (patients consulting) is 26 per 1000

- medical advice probably sought in only one in every ten cases of UTI

URINARY TRACT INFECTIONS

frequency

general practice

UTI in practice population of 2500

Annual new cases (incidence)	18
Annual patients consulting (prevalence)	65

district general hospital

DGH serving 250 000 persons (estimated)

Outpatient investigations	400

Admitted to hospital	125

high prevalence groups

- newborn
- preschool children
- schoolchildren
- women (20–60)
- pregnancy
- elderly (M < F)

prevalence rates of covert bacteriuria

- neonates (10 per 1000 : M < F)
- preschool (girls 8 per 1000)
- primary school (girls 16 per 1000; boys 0.4 per 1000)
- adult women (50 per 1000)

    rate rises with age and sexual activity

    one third of all women have an attack UTI at some time
- pregnancy (20–60 per 1000)
- adult men (5 per 1000)
- elderly (hospital patients) over 70

    males 200 per 1000

    females 250 per 1000

WHAT HAPPENS?

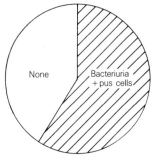

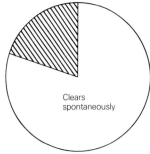

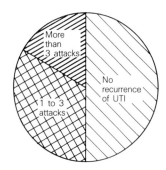

- unless there are associated abnormalities or diseases of the urinary tract the prognosis is good
- nine out of ten women with frequency/dysuria treat themselves, only one in ten consults her GP
- of those who do consult their GP

  39% have significant bacteriuria and pus cells

  8% have significant bacteriuria only

  12% have pus cells only

  41% have insignificant, equivocal or no bacteriuria or pus cells

- *uncomplicated UTI* – in 80% bacteriuria clears spontaneously without specific therapy

- of women presenting in general practice with *first attack of UTI* and followed up for 10 years

  half have no recurrences

  one third will have 1–3 attacks of UTI

  one fifth will have more than 3 attacks

  none will develop chronic renal failure

- recurrent bacteriuria in adult women does *not* lead to

  rise in BP

  rise in blood urea level

  kidney scarring

- *pregnancy*

  symptomatic UTI likely when covert bacteriuria present – *one third* develop acute pyelonephritis

  controlling bacteriuria reduces symptomatic UTI by 90%

WHAT TO DO?

- very common condition and most attacks of UTI in women are self-limiting and recover spontaneously
- in one half there is a single attack with no recurrence
- the problem cases are those with frequent recurrences and those in whom there may be an underlying organic condition
- which are the particular 'at-risk groups' that need to be picked out, investigated and treated?
- how can recurrences be prevented in those prone to such attacks?
- should population screening be carried out on selected groups?

diagnosis

history

- one half of patients with significant bacteriuria have no symptoms
- of the half with symptoms, approximately one half have 'bacterial cystitis' and one half have 'urethral syndrome' (abacterial cystitis)
- *acute pyelonephritis* is *uncommon* (less than one case a year in general practice)

cystitis

- frequency
- dysuria
- strangury
- suprapubic pain

acute pyelonephritis

- general   fever

                  rigors

                  nausea/vomiting

- local   loin pain → iliac fossae

                  frank haematuria

                  additional symptoms of cystitis may or may not be present

chronic pyelonephritis	<ul><li>not related to UTI unless some underlying pathology</li><li>often no symptoms</li><li>sometimes urinary symptoms</li></ul>

frequency

dysuria

lumbar ache

	• *uraemic symptoms* polyuria/polydipsia

lassitude

hiccoughs

drowsiness

twitching

diarrhoea

paraesthesiae
(neuropathy)

- *hypertensive symptoms*

throbbing occipital headache

epistaxis

coronary disease – angina

vascular – claudication

acute prostatitis	<ul><li>high fever</li><li>malaise</li><li>perineal pain</li><li>frequency</li><li>urgency</li><li>dysuria</li></ul>
chronic prostatitis	<ul><li>often asymptomatic</li><li>perineal or low back pain</li><li>dysuria</li></ul>

urethritis

- scalding urine
- strangury
- discharge

urinary tract infections in children

- *newborn* failure to gain weight

  apathy

  vomiting and diarrhoea

  abdominal distension

  occasionally convulsions

  fever (50% only)
- *childhood* frequency

  dysuria

  haematuria

  perineal or suprapubic pain

  acute abdominal pain and vomiting

examination

- some of the possible findings are shown in Figure 20.2
- *rectal examination* – tender prostate in acute prostatitis
- *vaginal examination* for pelvic inflammatory or neoplastic disease which might lead to urinary tract infection by direct spread of infection or by obstruction of ureter

investigations

UTI cannot be diagnosed on symptoms alone

urinalysis

- examination of the urine is only accurate if a very careful and uncontaminated midstream specimen of urine is collected and either sent straight to the laboratory or refrigerated until it is possible to dispatch to the laboratory

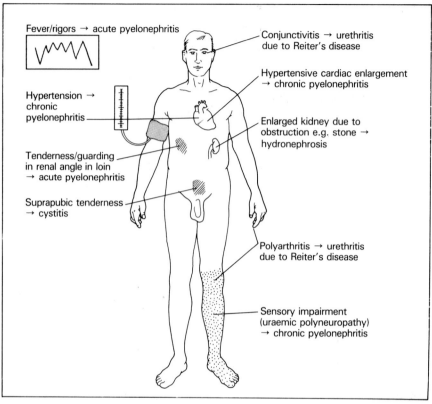

Fever/rigors → acute pyelonephritis

Conjunctivitis → urethritis
due to Reiter's disease

Hypertensive cardiac enlargement
→ chronic pyelonephritis

Hypertension →
chronic
pyelonephritis

Enlarged kidney due to
obstruction e.g. stone →
hydronephrosis

Tenderness/guarding
in renal angle in loin
→ acute pyelonephritis

Suprapubic tenderness
→ cystitis

Polyarthritis → urethritis
due to Reiter's disease

Sensory impairment
(uraemic polyneuropathy)
→ chronic pyelonephritis

Figure 20.2   *Possible findings in urinary tract infection*

- urinary findings

    cloudy and smelly

    acid in *E. coli* infections

    acute pyelonephritis

    pus cells > 2/high power field

    pus casts

    red cells

    epithelial cells

    pathogens   usual

    anaerobes

    ureaplasmas

    chlamydia

    L-phase bacteria

chronic pyelonephritis

    pus cells

    protein

    epithelial cells + +

cystitis

    pus cells

    red cells

    pathogens – *E. coli* most frequent in young women

- elderly patients may need catheterizing to obtain a urine specimen but this may introduce infection and great care is necessary to perform the procedure in as sterile a way as possible

- in difficult cases suprapubic aspiration of the bladder may be necessary to obtain a urine sample

- in suspected prostatitis, three samples of urine are collected with prostatic massage before the last specimen

localization of level of infection

- clinical features not always accurate since symptoms of lower urinary tract infection are often present with renal infection

- *indirect methods*

    detection of antibody coated urinary pathogens by fluorescent technique – correlates with renal parenchymal infection, e.g. acute pyelonephritis

    serum antibodies to a special protein (Tamm–Horsfall) develop with symptomatic acute pyelonephritis in children

    measurement of renal concentrating power – defect implies tubular involvement in kidney

    urinary enzyme excretion

white cell provocation test with intravenous pyrogen or steroid – substantial white cell excretion in the urine indicates latent pyelonephritis

- *direct methods*

    bladder catheterization and antibiotic wash-out – if pathogens are then found they must have come from ureters and kidneys

    individual ureteric catheterization and culture

    renal biopsy

radiology of the urinary tract

- main value is in detection of abnormalities amenable to surgical treatment
- indications

    young children of either sex

    men of all ages

    men and women with UTI if:

        associated bacteraemia

        ureteric colic

        passage of stones

        less common pathogens   pseudomonas

                                                    proteus

        repeated attacks of pyelonephritis affecting same kidney

- possible findings

    vesico-ureteric reflux in children

    obstructive nephropathy, e.g. stones

    chronic pyelonephritis (Figure 20.3)

    polycystic disease

    analgesic nephropathy   phenacetin

                                            aspirin

    atonic bladder in neurogenic disorders

    prostatic obstruction

    posterior urethral valve

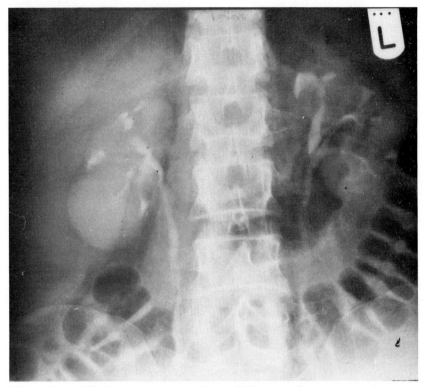

Figure 20.3 *IVP showing shrunken distorted kidneys with loss of cortical substance (especially in the right kidney) due to chronic pyelonephritis*

- *types of X-ray*

    intravenous pyelogram

    retrograde pyelogram

    micturating cystogram – especially for reflux

differential diagnosis of acute pyelonephritis

acute appendicitis

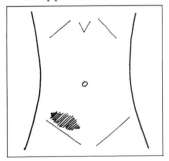

- only low-grade fever
- no loin tenderness
- rebound tenderness present
- pyuria absent

acute cholecystitis

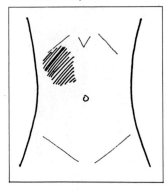

- right hypochondriac pain radiating to shoulder
- gallstone colic
- jaundice
- Murphy's sign present
- pyuria absent
- tests help   bilirubin ↑

                           alkaline phosphatase ↑

                           X-ray – opaque stone

                           cholecystogram

                           ultrasound

                           i.v. cholangiogram

acute salpingitis

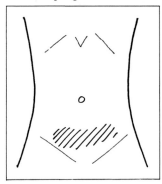

- predisposing factors

      septic abortion

      recent delivery

      V.D.

- rebound pelvic tenderness
- vaginal discharge
- pain p.v. on moving cervix
- mass in pelvis p.v.

acute diverticulitis

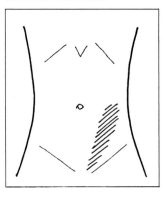

- long history abdominal pain
- diarrhoea, rectal bleeding common
- mass in LIF
- p.v. – mass in Pouch of Douglas
- tests   sigmoidoscopy

             barium enema

diaphragmatic pleurisy	• pain worse on coughing/deep breathing
	• associated cough and phlegm of underlying pneumonia
	• abnormal physical signs in chest
	• no urinary abnormalities – no pus cells/organisms
	• tests – chest X-ray
perinephric abscess	• urinary symptoms absent
	• oedema in loin
	• severe constitutional symptoms
	• may be recent purulent infection elsewhere, e.g. carbuncle
	• no pus cells/pathogens in urine
	• tests high white cell count
	ultrasound
	CT scan

differential diagnosis of chronic pyelonephritis

renal tuberculosis	• tuberculosis elsewhere
	• general malaise
	fever
	lassitude
	weight loss
	• recurrent haematuria prominent
	• tests
	urine – sterile pyuria
	culture of ureteric urine for TB
	i.v.p. may help
	cystoscopy – may show tubercles

carcinoma

bladder
- may be aniline dye worker
- lone haematuria common
- urinary obstruction may occur
- tests   i.v.p.
          cystoscopy and biopsy

prostate
- urethral obstruction
  difficulty in micturition
  poor urinary stream
  anuria may occur
  overflow incontinence may occur
  haematuria
  bone pain from metastases
    stony hard prostate
    distended bladder
  tests
    i.v.p. – prostatic obstruction
    raised acid phosphatase
    urethroscopy and biopsy
    X-ray spine/pelvis – metastases

kidney
- haematuria most frequent symptom
- renal colic due to blood clot
- discomfort in loin
- long-continued fever (P.U.O.)
- examination – renal mass
- tests   blood count →polycythaemia
          i.v.p.
          ultrasound
          CT scan
          angiography

management of clinical types

women

- *women with infrequent attacks*
  - general advice
    - fluids +
    - genital toilet
    - frequent passing of urine
  - test urine
  - if symptoms persist → antibacterial therapy
    - single dose
      - amoxycillin 3 g
      - co-trimoxazole (Septrin) 2.88 g
      - kanamycin 0.5 g i.m.
      - cephamandole 1 gm
    - 5–7 days
      - sulphonamide
      - nitrofurantoin (Furadantin)
      - nalidixic acid (Negram)
- *women with frequent attacks*
  - enquire for precipitating cause
  - examine for possible abnormalities (GU)
    - renal stone
    - other obstruction
  - test urine
  - consider i.v.p., cystoscopy
  - general advice
  - consider prophylactic chemotherapy
    - ampicillin
    - amoxycillin
    - nitrofurantoin
    - nalidixic acid
    - cephalosporins

length of courses

    3–6 weeks

    6 weeks – 6 months

review antibiotic monthly after urine tests

- *acute pyelonephritis*

treat acute attack intensively with antibiotics

may need hospital admission

fully investigate after infection settles for any underlying organic disease, e.g. stones

- *pregnancy*

repeated checks for UTI

treat bacteriuria or UTI with antibiotic/ chemotherapy – amoxycillin, sulphonamides and nitrofurantoin can all be used safely in early pregnancy

treat for 1 week : follow-up regularly and if infection recurs treat for longer periods

men

- always consider underlying cause – especially bladder neck obstruction (prostatic enlargement)

- chronic bacterial prostatitis

co-trimoxazole best

12-week course

only one third cured

- always investigate fully even after 1st attack

covert bacteriuria

- *covert bacteriuria in non-pregnant women with normal urinary tract*

no need to treat

follow-up for any signs of renal damage which is unlikely

- *covert bacteriuria with underlying organic disease of urinary tract*

  associated with

  renal stones

  analgesic nephropathy

  vesico-ureteric reflux

  effective chemotherapy mandatory to avoid further damage

  prolonged chemotherapy often necessary

urinary infection with obstruction

- medical/surgical emergency
- effective chemotherapy essential
- urgent surgery to relieve obstruction

children

- urinalysis in all children with any possible symptoms relating to UTI

  non-thriving

  recurrent fevers

  recurring abdominal pains

  enuresis

  frequency/dysuria

- if UTI confirmed, then investigate fully even after first attack

risks of drug treatment in renal failure

- nitrofurantoin (Furadantin), nalidixic acid

  ineffective

  may be toxic, e.g. neuropathy with Furadantin

- tetracycline – may precipitate uraemia
- co-trimoxazole

  impairs renal function

  use reduced dose

- aminoglycosides (e.g. gentamicin)

  toxic

  reduce dose
- diuretics – potentiate toxicity of aminoglycosides and cephalosporins

screening

- random mass population screening for covert bacteriuria is not cost-effective
- possible justification in selected at-risk groups

  pregnancy

  neonates

  diabetics

Useful practical points

- UTI may be present without any symptom of frequency/dysuria
- suspect UTI in vague real illness in children and in elderly
- most prevalent in women 20–60 and here the problems are unfortunate ladies with recurring UTI – for whom the many treatments and advice suggested denote no single cause or effective treatment
- many attacks in adult women settle with placebos
- antibiotics and chemotherapy should be used selectively and with discrimination
- think of UTI in non-thriving infants and in girls with recurring abdominal symptoms, but few of these are caused by UTI
- in *men* UTI is generally secondary to some primary cause such as bladder neck obstruction, sexually transmitted diseases, calculi etc
- the most problematical group, adult women with frequent UTI attacks, eventually cease attacks after 55–60

---

21 PREGNANCY

WHAT IS IT?

- pregnancy is not a disease
- pregnancy is a normal state of human life and reproduction
- data on pregnancy show how it may be used to create a profile of quality and quantity of care

WHAT AND HOW MUCH?

annual birth rates

- *annual birth rates per 1000 population.* The birth rates in UK since World War II reached a peak in 1964 and have since been declining

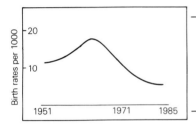

1951	15.7
1961	17.8
1964	18.7
1971	16.0
1981	12.8
1983	12.7

Data : ref 44

- the birth rate in 1983 meant 700 000 births or 25 per GP.

total fertility rates

- average number of children that would be born per woman if women experienced the age-specific fertility rates during their child-bearing life span

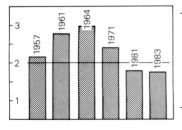

1951	2.16
1961	2.78
1964	2.93
1971	2.40
1981	1.79
1983	1.75

Data : ref.44

- these rates mean that since 1981 two parents were producing fewer than two children, so population is likely to fall, if such rates continue

legal abortions

In 1983, in addition to the 700 000 births there were 140 000 legal abortions in British residents, or one in six of all pregnancies (excluding natural abortions)[44]

WHO?

age of mother

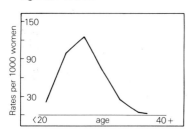

- UK birth rates per 1000 women in the age groups in 1983

Age	All women 15–45	< 20	20–	25–	30–	35–	40–45
Rates per 1000 women	59.7	26.9	98.5	126.4	71.5	23.1	4.8

place of birth of mother

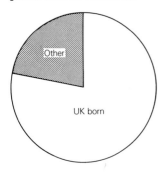

- United Kingdom   88.0
- Irish Republic and 'old Commonwealth'   1.4
- 'new Commonwealth'   7.7
- other countries   2.9

                  ————

                  100

                  ————

(Data : ref 44)

WHERE BORN?

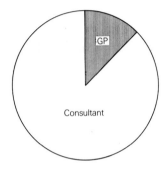

% born in hospital

- almost all births in UK now take place in hospitals

	1959	1971	1981
Hospital	65%	88%	98.7%
Home	35%	12%	1.3%

place of births

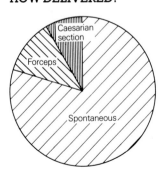

GP

Consultant

- of births taking place in *hospitals* (1981)

consultant units	87.5%
GP beds in consultant units	5.2%
GP – separate units	6.0%
	98.7%

- *GPs* are *responsible* for 12.5% of deliveries (hospital + home)

WHO CARES?

antenatal care

- GPs are involved in shared care in over 75% of pregnancies

delivery

- midwives deliver 82% of all births without medical assistance[45]

HOW DELIVERED?

Caesarian section

Forceps

Spontaneous

spontaneous (breech 3%)	80%
episiotomy	45%
forceps	12%
caesarean section	8%
induced	25%
accelerated	18%
epidural	13%

Data : ref. 45

WHAT OUTCOMES?

- pregnancies are becoming safer

mother

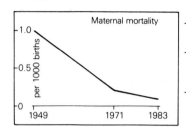

- maternal mortality in UK has fallen tenfold since 1949

	1949	1971	1983
Maternal mortality per 1000 births	1.0	0.17	0.10

child

- indices of safety for infants have improved

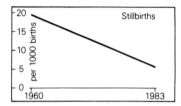

	1960	1983	
Stillbirths	19.5	5.7	per 1000 live & stillbirths
Early neonatal (in first week)	13.2	4.6	per 1000 live births
Infant mortality (in first year)	21.6	10.0	

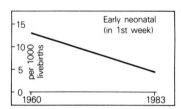

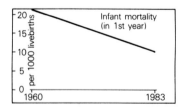

Useful practical points

- birth rates have been falling since 1964
- UK population is not being replaced by present fertility rates
- one in six of all births end by legal abortion (excluding natural abortions)
- highest birth rate at 25–30 years
- 98.7% of births now take place in hospital
- GPs responsible for care of 12.5% actual births
- GPs involved in over 75% of antenatal care
- midwives deliver 82% of babies unaided
- all indices of outcome are improving

22   CANCERS

WHAT ARE THEY?

uncontrolled cell growth +
invasion of tissues
metastases
metabolic disturbances
death

- cancer is not a single disease
- cancer is a body process as are 'inflammation' or 'atheroma'
- the main features are abnormal growth of abnormal cells – cells which are out of control, invade adjacent tissues, metastasize to distant parts of the body and in some produce major metabolic and other disturbances and death
- the clinical manifestations of cancers depend on the types of cells involved, on the organs affected and on other individual factors

WHO, WHEN AND WHERE?

age incidence

overall most cancers are age related with an incidence that increases with age but there are varieties that are most frequent in childhood or in middle age

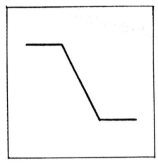

Wilms'

retinoblastoma

neuroblastoma

acute leukaemias

osteogenic sarcoma

} childhood

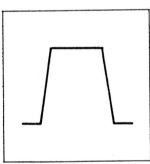

testicular

chorioepithelioma

cervix

uterine body

ovary

Hodgkin's

} middle age

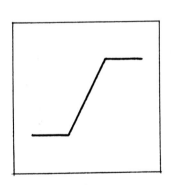

lung

stomach

large bowel

bladder

prostate

larynx

breast

oesophagus

pancreas

} aged

sex/sites

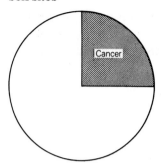

- In 1981 – 148 710 *deaths* from cancer in UK (25% of all deaths)
- M : F = 1.4 : 1

sites in cancer deaths

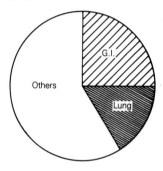

sites in cancer deaths (%)

gastrointestinal tract	25
lung	16
breast	15
renal/bladder/prostate	13
uterus/ovaries	9
skin	9
others	13
	100

males

- *males* (deaths from cancers, 1981)

brain	1420
oesophagus	2580
lung	30 000
stomach	7500
pancreas	3340
colon	5060
rectum	3640
bladder	3300
prostate	5750
leukaemia	2050
others	14 000
	78 640

females

- *females* (deaths from cancers, 1981)

oesophagus	1910
lung	9730
breast	14 000
stomach	4960
pancreas	3160
colon	6800
rectum	3090
ovary	4140
cervix	2260
leukaemia	1720
others	17 300
	69 070

Data : ref. 46

mortality rates from cancer

- in UK *one quarter of all deaths* are from cancers

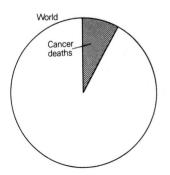

- in the world *only 8% of all deaths* are from cancers
- cancers are more likely to be causes of death in developed than developing countries

- annual incidence (new cases): 3.5 per 1000

  annual death rate (from cancers) : 2.5 per 1000

general practice

- annual incidence (new cases) of cancers in population of 2500

All cancers	10
Lung	3
Breast	2
Skin	1

Less than 1 per year	*per years*
Prostate	4 in 5
Stomach	1 in 2
Colon	1 in 2
Cervix	2 in 5
Cervix *in situ*	1 in 3
Rectum	1 in 3
Ovary	1 in 3
Uterus (body)	1 in 4
Bladder	1 in 4
Pancreas	1 in 5
Leukaemia (all types)	1 in 5
Larynx	1 in 10
Brain	1 in 10
Oesophagus	1 in 12
Hodgkin's	1 in 15
Thyroid	1 in 15
Testis	1 in 15
Melanoma	1 in 20

district general hospital

- almost 150 000 persons die each year from cancers and most die in hospitals after long suffering and treatment

- in addition the DGH is involved in diagnosis and management in the pre-terminal stages and since there is a 36% 5-year survival rate, the numbers involved are appreciable and spread over many departments

DGH serving 250 000 population

Annual referrals for all cancers	1000

Annual numbers of types of cancers	
Lung	350
Breast	250
Skin	100
Prostate	85
Stomach	50
Colon	50
Cervix	40
Cervix *in situ*	35
Rectum	35
Ovary	35
Uterus body	25
Bladder	25
Pancreas	20
Leukaemia	20
Larynx	10
Brain	10
Oesophagus	8
Hodgkin's	6
Thyroid	6
Testis	6
Melanoma	2

WHAT HAPPENS?

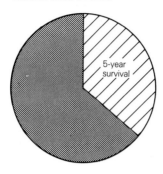

- for all cancers the 5-year+ survival rate is 36%
- the *survival rates* vary with the cancer sites

Cancer	5-year + survival (%)
Skin	95
(Melanoma)	(50)
Chorioepithelioma	80
Testis	67
Uterus (body)	67
Larynx	60
Breast	57
Hodgkin's	57
Cervix	54
Bladder	50
Prostate	36
Kidney	34
Rectum	32
Lymphosarcoma	31
Colon	30
Leukaemia	25
Ovary	25
Oesophagus	7
Stomach	7
Lung	7
Pancreas	3
All cancers	36

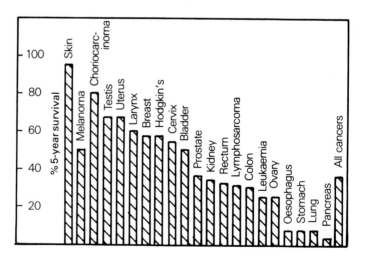

WHAT TO DO?

issues

- with a 36% 5-year survival, the results of therapy are poor for many cancer patients and even with technological advances these rates are unlikely to be much improved

- the main hopes in the future are in *prevention*

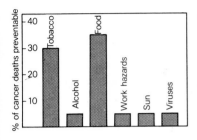

- the causes of cancer are uncertain but some *risk factors* can be defined, such as cigarette smoking, alcohol, diets and food, hazards at work, radiation and sunlight and viruses

- Doll and Peto (1982)[47] have quantified definite and possible preventable cancer deaths

- *early diagnosis* is the other hope for improving survival as the earlier that many cancers are treated the better the prognosis

diagnosis of cancer

the clinical diagnosis of cancer is based on

- local effects
- metastatic effects
- systemic effects

local effects

- visible/palpable mass
  - breast lump
  - skin lump
  - bony lump
  - muscle lump
  - enlarged glands
- invasion and tissue destruction
  - organ dysfunction
  - pain
    - nerve infiltration
      - brachial plexus (cancer lung, breast)
      - sacral plexus (cancer cervix, rectum)
      - paraspinal (cancer pancreas)
      - referred – shoulder, hip, knee

bleeding

    cancer lung → haemoptysis

    cancer stomach → haematemesis

    cancer colon → rectal bleed

    kidney/bladder cancer → haematuria

- obstruction

    vascular (veins/lympatics) → oedema

    bronchi → breathlessness

    oesophagus → dysphagia

    ureter → renal (loin) pain

    biliary tract → jaundice

metastatic effects

- lung →

    cough

    breathlessness

    haemoptysis

- brain →

    fit

    focal neurological disturbance

    raised intracranial pressure →

        headache

        vomiting

        papilloedema

- liver → pain due to distension

- bone →

    pain

    fractures

systemic effects

constitutional

- cachexia
   - increased metabolic rate in cancer
   - malnutrition   anorexia
     - GI obstruction
     - pancreatic deficiency
     - lack of bile
- weight loss
   - hypermetabolic state
   - inadequate calorie intake
- anorexia? due to products of malignancy
- fever especially   Hodgkin's disease
   - lymphoma
   - cancer kidney
   - hepatic metastases

para-neoplastic syndromes

- *skin*
   - acanthosis nigricans
     - carcinoma stomach
     - other adenocarcinomas
   - dermatomyositis
     - cancer lung (commonest)
     - breast cancer
     - GI tract cancer
     - GU tract cancer
   - flushing – argentaffin tumours
     - bowel
     - lung
   - pigmentation – oat cell cancer lung (ACTH/MSH)

- *neuromuscular*

    Eaton–Lambert syndrome – cancer lung

    polyneuropathy

    cerebellar degeneration

    dementia due to leukoencephalopathy

    'motor neurone disease' syndrome

- *vascular*

    venous thrombosis especially cancer
    pancreas

    marantic endocarditis

- *metabolic/hormonal*

    Cushing's syndrome – cancer lung

    excessive antidiuretic hormone

    gynaecomastia – testicular tumours

    diarrhoea – islet cell tumour

    hypoglycaemia – pancreatic tumour

    hypercalcaemia   myeloma

                           cancer breast

                           cancer kidney

                           cancer lung

    hypocalcaemia – cancer prostate with
    metastases

- *renal*

    nephrotic syndrome

        myeloma/amyloid

        Hodgkin's disease

        cancer colon

    proximal tubular defect – acute monocytic
    leukaemia

blood	• anaemia
	malignancy
	blood loss, e.g. cancer colon
	haemolytic – lymphoma
	leuko-erythroblastic – marrow infiltration
	red cell aplasia – thymoma

blood
- anaemia
  - malignancy
  - blood loss, e.g. cancer colon
  - haemolytic – lymphoma
  - leuko-erythroblastic – marrow infiltration
  - red cell aplasia – thymoma
- erythrocytosis   cancer kidney
  - Wilms' tumour
  - cerebellar tumour
- eosinophilia   cancer lung
  - Hodgkin's disease
- thrombocytopenia immune reaction
  - hypersplenism
  - Hodgkin's
  - lymphoma
- disseminated intravascular coagulation

skeleton
- clubbing of fingers → cancer lung
- hypertrophic pulmonary osteoarthropathy → cancer lung

symptoms and signs of specific cancers

lung
- probably commonest cancer of all
  clinical features in Figure 22.1

colon/rectum
- see Figure 22.2

stomach
- see Figure 22.3

pancreas
- see Figure 22.4

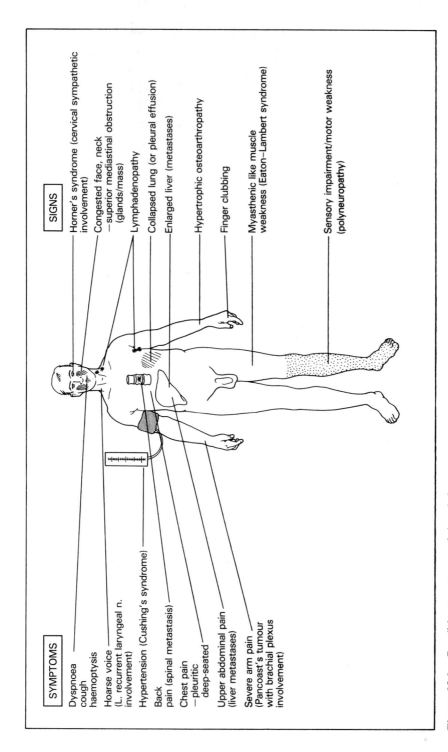

Figure 22.1 *Possible symptoms and signs in lung cancer*

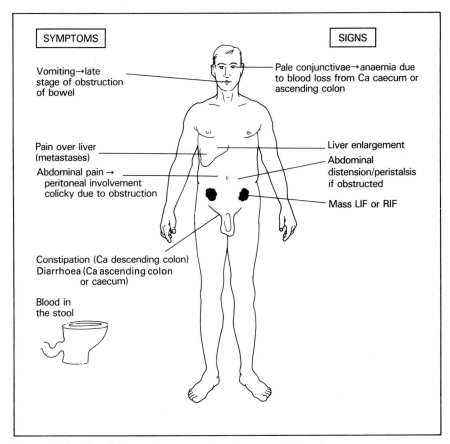

Figure 22.2 *Possible symptoms and signs in cancer of the colon*

breast

- symptoms
    - lump in breast
    - discharge from nipple
    - severe back pain (metastasis)
- signs
    - lump in breast
    - 'orange-peel' skin
    - axillary lymphadenopathy

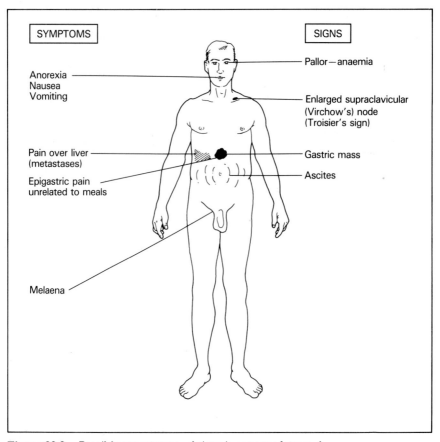

Figure 22.3   *Possible symptoms and signs in cancer of stomach*

uterus

- symptoms
    abnormal vaginal bleeding
    abdominal swelling (ascites)
    severe leg pain (sacral plexus infiltration)
    pelvic pain
- signs
    cervical mass/ulcer p.v.
    ascites (peritoneal involvement)

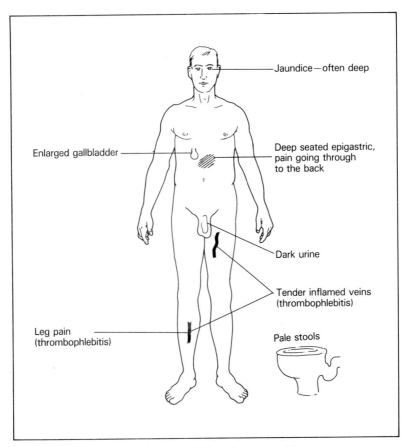

Figure 22.4 *Possible symptoms and signs in cancer of the pancreas*

prostate

- symptoms
  - dysuria
  - haematuria
  - bone pain especially spine
- signs
  - enlarged hard prostate p.r.
  - spinal tenderness

ovary

- symptoms
  - nausea, vomiting
  - pelvic pain
  - abdominal swelling (ascites)
  - breathlessness (pleural effusion)
- signs
  - ovarian mass p.v.
  - ascites
  - pleural effusion (Meigs's syndrome)

testis

- symptoms
  - pain in testis
  - swelling in testis
- signs
  - testicular mass
  - lymphadenopathy grown
  - gynaecomastia

myeloma

- symptoms
  - of anaemia
  - bone pain
  - renal colic/failure
  - susceptible to infection
  - lethargy/drowsiness (hypercalcaemia)
  - headache/dizziness (hyperviscosity)
- signs
  - tender bones especially vertebrae
  - retinopathy (hyperviscosity)
  - anaemia
  - oedema/ascites (nephrotic syndrome due to amyloidosis)

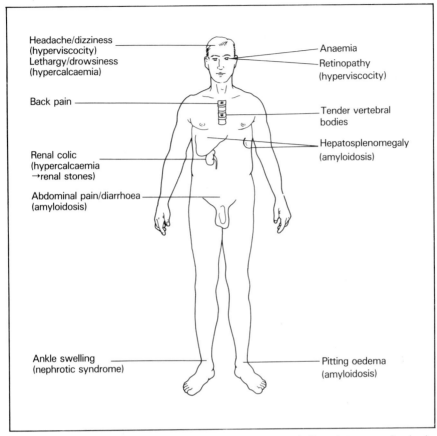

Headache/dizziness
(hyperviscocity)
Lethargy/drowsiness
(hypercalcaemia)

Anaemia

Retinopathy
(hyperviscocity)

Back pain

Tender vertebral
bodies

Hepatosplenomegaly
(amyloidosis)

Renal colic
(hypercalcaemia
→renal stones)

Abdominal pain/diarrhoea
(amyloidosis)

Ankle swelling
(nephrotic syndrome)

Pitting oedema
(amyloidosis)

Figure 22.5 *Possible symptoms and signs in myelomatosis ('renal stones and pains in bones')*

Hodgkin's disease	● see Figure 22.6
hepatobiliary	● symptoms
	repeated biliary colic
	pain right hypochondrium
	jaundice
	● signs
	jaundice
	palpable gallbladder
	liver enlargement

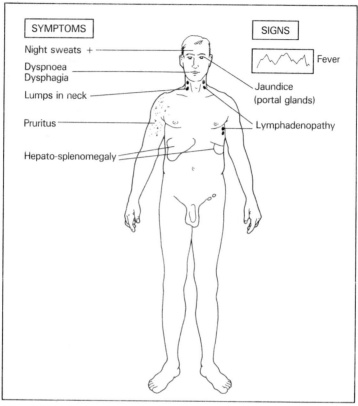

Figure 22.6   *Possible symptoms and signs in Hodgkin's disease*

kidney

- symptoms
  - loin pain
  - haematuria
  - altered mental state (hypercalcaemia)
- sign
  - renal mass

brain

- symptoms
  - headache
  - vomiting
  - fits

CANCERS

investigations in cancer　　　the function of investigations in cancer is to

- establish the diagnosis
- decide whether the tumour is benign or malignant
- determine degree of malignancy with particular reference to

  prognosis

  response to radiotherapy or chemotherapy

tests

types　　　　　　　　types of tests

- simple non-invasive, e.g. X-rays
- special tests – often invasive
- histology tests

  surgical biopsy

  cytology　　　　　sputum

  　　　　　　　　　pleural fluid

  　　　　　　　　　ascitic fluid

  　　　　　　　　　cervical smears

  needle aspiration　breast

  　　　　　　　　　subcutaneous

  　　　　　　　　　lung

  　　　　　　　　　liver

application　　　　　application of these tests to the diagnosis of specific cancers is shown in Table 22.1

laboratory　　　　　simple laboratory tests which are of special value in the diagnosis of cancer include

- hypercalcaemia

  multiple myeloma

  carcinoma metastases especially

  　　lung

  　　breast

  　　kidney

Table 22.1 – *Diagnostic tests in cancer*

Cancer	Simple	Special	Histology
lung			
primary	chest X-ray tomogram	bronchoscopy	sputum bronchoscopy pleural biopsy lung biopsy
metastases	I.V.P. barium studies	thyroid scan mammogram	lung biopsy
gastrointestinal			
stomach	barium meal	gastroscopy carcinoembryonic antigen	gastroscopic biopsy
colon	barium enema faecal occult blood I.V.P.	sigmoidoscopy colonoscopy carcinoembryonic antigen	biopsy through 'scope
pancreas	ultrasound I.V. cholangiogram	ERCP isotope scan arteriogram CT scan carcinoembryonic antigen	duodenal aspiration ERCP biopsy laparotomy
oesophasgus	chest X-ray barium swallow	oesophagoscopy bronchoscopy mediastinoscopy CT scan	'scope biopsy
gallbladder	ultrasound cholecystogram I.V. cholangiogram	isotope scan ERCP CT scan α-fetoprotein carcinoembryonic antigen	ERCP biopsy laparotomy
liver – single	ultrasound	isotope scan peritoneoscopy arteriogram α-fetoprotein	percutaneous biopsy peritoneoscopy biopsy laparotomy
liver – metastases	chest X-ray barium series ultrasound	mammogram isotope scan	percutaneous biopsy peritoneoscopy biopsy laparotomy
breast	X-ray bones	mammogram mammary thermogram bone scan oestrogen/progesterone receptors	direct biopsy needle biopsy

Cancer	Simple	Special	Histology
genito-urinary prostate	I.V.P serum acid phosphatase X-ray bones	bone scan	needle biopsy bone marrow
kidney	urine for red cells I.V.P. ultrasound	arteriogram venography – inferior cava erythropoietin level	urine ureteral drainage laparotomy
bladder	urine for red cells I.V.P.	cystoscopy	'scope biopsy
uterus	I.V.P.	colposcopy	Papanicolaou smear D&C laparotomy
ovary	ultrasound barium enema I.V.P	oestrogen/ progesterone receptors	peritoneoscopy laparotomy
testis	ultrasound	thermography α-fetoprotein carcinoembryonic antigen gonadotrophin excretion	surgical
lymphoma (& Hodgkin's)	chest X-ray (glands) abdo X-ray (spleen) ultrasound I.V.P blood count (hypersplenism)	isotope scan liver/spleen lymphangiogram CT scan venogram – inferior vena cava	excisional biopsy bone marrow peritoneoscopy laparotomy
leukaemia	blood count	Philadelphia chromosome (chronic myeloid leukaemia) leukocyte alkaline phosphatase	bone marrow
brain tumours	X-ray skull E.E.G.	CT scan arteriography	burr biopsy direct biopsy

- hypocalcaemia

    carcinoma prostate with extensive metastases

- hypoglycaemia

    islet cell tumour of pancreas

    retroperitoneal sarcoma

    hepatoma

- hyperglycaemia

    Cushing's syndrome due to oat-cell carcinoma of lung

- blood urea ↑

    urinary obstruction

    cancer cervix

    other pelvic tumours

    renal stones

    calcium – hypercalcaemic neoplasm

    uric acid

    leukaemias

    other myelo- or lymphoproliferative neoplasms

- liver function tests especially bilirubin and alkaline phosphatase – abnormal in biliary obstruction

    cancer gallbladder

    cancer Ampulla of Vater

    cancer pancreas

- serum proteins/immunoglobulins – multiple myeloma

- acid phosphatase – cancer prostate

tumour markers	these are chemical products produced by neoplastic cells and their presence acts as a 'marker' for the tumour

- carcinoembryonic antigen

  cancer rectum/colon

  other cancer GI tract

  non-malignant conditions

  - cirrhosis
  - diabetes
  - inflammatory bowel disease
  - pancreatitis

- α-fetoprotein

  cancer liver

  cancer testis/ovary

  cancer pancreas

  cancer lung

  cancer stomach/colon

  non-malignant conditions from amniotic fluid

  - spina bifida
  - anencephaly

- chorionic gonadotrophin

  cancer testis/ovary

  GI cancer   stomach

                   pancreas

                   liver

- polypeptides

  insulin/gastrin – islet cell tumour

  ACTH – oat-cell cancer lung

  ADH – oat-cell cancer lung

  calcitonin – oat-cell cancer lung

  5-HIAA – carcinoid syndrome

early diagnosis/screening

early diagnostic/screening measures

- cervical cytology
- breast examination
- occult blood in stools
- endoscopy of colon/rectum
- chest radiography

N.B. there is uncertainty over cost effectiveness of such national exercises

early diagnosis also depends on clinical acumen and investigating possible clinical danger signals:

- risk factors

  positive family history

  personal habits   tobacco

                       alcohol

                       excessive sun

  occupation   asbestos contact

                       chromium work

                       aniline dyes

- non-specific symptoms

  fatigue

  unexplained weight loss

  unusual persistent pain

  unexplained headache

  change in bowel habits

  persistent cough

  hoarseness of voice

- lab results

  unexplained

  anaemia

  thrombocytopenia

  hypercalcaemia

  high ESR

TREATMENT OF CANCER   objectives

- cure – may be based on 5–10 years survival
- prolongation and improvement of the quality of life
- palliation only

types of treatment available

- surgery
- radiotherapy
- chemotherapy/hormones
- any combination

factors influencing choice of treatment

- what is the aim

    to cure

    to improve

    to palliate

- staging of growth (TNM)

    local size (T)

    regional nodes (N)

    distant metastases (M)

- localized disease

    surgery

    radiotherapy

- disseminated

    chemotherapy

    hormones

- age of patient

management of cancers ranges from possible 'cures' for some types and relief and palliation for all

surgery

- removal of localized disease
- reduce tumour bulk to facilitate subsequent radio/chemotherapy, e.g.

    ovarian cancer

    large abdominal lymphoma

- bypass intestinal obstruction from cancer
- occasionally resection pulmonary metastases e.g. from
    - cancer testis/ovary
    - sarcomas

radiotherapy

- teletherapy most frequent
    - Cobalt^{60}
    - linear accelerator
- brachytherapy sometimes (enclosed isotope)
    - Caesium^{137} implantation – cancer cervix
    - Iridium^{192} – cancer breast
- killing of tumour cells related to dose
- indications
    - cure
        - Hodgkin's disease
        - other lymphomas
        - cancer cervix
        - cancer larynx
        - cancer prostate
        - cancer thyroid
        - seminoma
        - some skin cancer
    - relieve pain, e.g. myeloma in vertebra
    - prevent fractures from bony metastases
    - relieve obstruction
        - bronchus
        - GI tract
        - lymphatics
        - veins

side-effects

early   erythema/skin burns

nausea/vomiting

diarrhoea

alopecia

bone marrow suppression

late   radiation pneumonitis

stenosis in bowel

transverse myelitis

sterility

leukaemia

other carcinoma

chemotherapy

- types of drugs and indications are shown in Table 22.2
- response

  cure

      acute lymphoblastic leukaemia

      Burkitt's lymphoma

      Hodgkin's disease

      Wilms' tumour

      teratoma of testis

      choriocarcinoma

  remission

      cancer breast

      cancer ovary

      cancer lung (oat-cell)

      lymphoma (non-Hodgkin's)

      chronic lymphatic leukaemia

      acute myeloid leukaemia

      medulloblastoma

  partial remission

      cancer stomach

Table 22.2 *Chemotherapy of cancer*

Class of drug	Specific drug	Cancer indication
Alkylating	nitrogen mustard cyclophosphamide busulphan melphalan chlorambucil thiotepa	leukaemia myeloma lymphoma
Antimetabolite	methotrexate 6-mercaptopurine 6-thioguanine 5-fluorouracil cytosine aribinoside	leukaemia Ca breast Ca GI tract
Antibiotic	actinomycin-D adriamycin daunorubicin bleomycin mitomycin-C	Wilms' tumour Ca testis lymphoma
Plant alkaloids	vincristine vinblastine VP 16–213 VM 26	leukaemia lymphoma Ca testis
Nitrosoureas	BCNU CCNU methyl CCNU streptozotocin	lymphoma brain tumours
Miscellaneous	CIS platinum hydroxyurea methyl hydrazine procarbazine	Ca testis/ovary leukaemia lymphoma Ca lung

myeloma

cancer bladder

cancer pancreas

cancer thyroid

sarcoma

resistant

squamous cell cancer lung

cancer oesophagus

cancer colon

melanoma

- side-effects

  gastrointestinal   mouth ulcers

                                 nausea/vomiting

                                 diarrhoea

  alopecia   adriamycin

                      cyclophosphamide

  stunted growth in children

  amenorrhoea

  sterility

  heart failure – adriamycin

  renal failure – cisplatinum

  pulmonary fibrosis – bleomycin

  neuropathy – vinca alkaloids

  secondary malignancy, e.g. acute leukaemia with alkylating agents

- combination of drugs more likely to induce remission

  nitrogen mustard, vincristine, procarbazine, prednisolone

  indications

     leukaemia

     Hodgkin's disease

     cancer breast, ovary, lung, testis

  21-day cycles produce least marrow depression – always monitor blood count

endocrine treatment

- may be effective in tumours under hormonal control

  breast

  prostate

  uterus

  thyroid

- removal of hormones for cancer breast

    aminoglutethamide – 'chemical' adrenalectomy

    adrenalectomy

    oophorectomy

    tamoxifen – blocks oestrogen

- administration of hormones

    androgens – cancer breast and metastases

    oestrogens – cancer prostate

    progesterone – cancer uterus with metastases

    thyroxine – cancer thyroid

- side-effects

    tamoxifen – drowsiness

    aminoglutethamide   rashes

    drowsiness

    depression

    oestrogens – fluid retention and heart failure in elderly man with cancer prostate

terminal care

- essential when treatment is no longer effective in controlling tumour growth and patient is entering terminal phase of illness

- anxieties of the dying patient

    pain

    isolation/loneliness

    dependence on others

    loss of dignity

    consequences for dependents

    act of dying

    life after death

- requirements
  - control of pain from
    - nerve compression
    - bony metastases
    - invasion of organs
    - obstruction of organs
  - measures
    - analgesics
      - aspirin/codeine
      - dextromoramide
      - buprenorphine
      - netopam
      - phenazocine
      - morphine
      - heroin
    - nerve blocks
    - cordotomy
    - other
      - hypnosis
      - acupuncture
  - control nausea/vomiting
    - metoclopromide
    - other antiemetics
  - measures for constipation
  - support until death – no isolation
  - consider spiritual as well as physical support
- facilities available
  - home – support required from
    - family
    - primary care team
    - community resources
    - special nurses (Macmillan)
    - day centre
  - hospice
  - hospital

- *should the doctor tell the patient?*

  always try to find enough time to talk to the patient

  find out what the patient really wants to know

  never tell a deliberate untruth though it may not be appropriate to tell the whole truth

  most patients are bound to find out sometime

  if he doesn't know he cannot use the remaining precious time properly

  it imposes a severe burden on the family if the patient doesn't know

  he may wish to prepare for the 'after-life' and will need spiritual, as well as medical, help

---

Useful practical points

- a lump in the breast should always be regarded as malignant until proved otherwise
- an underlying bronchial carcinoma should be considered in any slowly-resolving pneumonia in a middle-aged or elderly patient
- carcinoma of the lung cannot be excluded until bronchoscopy has been carried out, and even then about one third of tumours are missed
- it is unwise to attribute recent bleeding in a middle-aged patient to piles until carcinoma of the colon is excluded by sigmoidoscopy and barium enema
- patients with anxiety syndromes can also develop organic disease, e.g. cancer of the oesophagus in globus hystericus and cancer of the colon in a patient with irritable bowel syndrome
- CT scanning can detect 95% of all brain tumours – it supersedes all other tests
- remember the possibility of associated phaeochromocytoma in a patient with thyroid cancer
- rapid deterioration in a patient with cirrhosis can be due to the development of carcinoma of the liver

References

1. Fry, J. (1985). *Common Diseases*. 4th Edn. (Lancaster: MTP Press)

2. Kannel, W. B. and Dawber, T. R. (1974). *Br. J. Hosp. Med.*, **11**, 508

3. Rajala, S. *et al.* (1983). *Lancet*, **2**, 520–1

4. Lindholm, L. *et al.* (1983). *Lancet*, **2**, 745–6

5. Gill, J. S. and Beevers, D. G. (1983). 1–16 *Cardiology in Practice* (London)

6. Australian Therapeutic Trial on Untreated Mild Hypertension (1982). *Lancet*, **1**, 185–91

7. Peach, H. and Heller, R. F. (1984). *Epidemiology of Common Diseases*. (London: Heinemann)

8. Office of Health Economics (1982). *Coronary Heart Disease*. (London: OHE)

9. Rose, G. (1981). *Br. Med. J.*, **1**, 1847–51

10. Colling, A. (1977). *Coronary Care in the Community*. (London: Croom Helm)

11. Warlow, C. P. (1983). *Br. Med. J.*, **287**, 713–17

12. Black, D. G. *et al.* (1984). *Br. Med. J.*, **2**, 156–9

13. Moser, M. (1984), *J. Public Health Policy*, **5**, 228–37

14. Pearson, R. S. B. (1958). *Allergologica*, **12**, 227–9

15. Office of Health Economics. (1977). *Preventing Bronchitis*. (London: OHE)

16. Crean, G. P. (1984). *Peptic Ulcer*. (Update Seminar Series, ed. Lancaster-Smith, M.) (London: Update)

17. Sircus, W. (1984). *Peptic Ulceration and its Management*. (Greenford, Mddx.: Glaxo Laboratories)

18. Langman, M. J. S. and Cooke, A. R. (1976). Gastric and duodenal ulcer and their associated diseases. *Lancet*, **1**, 680–3

19. Avery Jones, F. (1957). Clinical and social problems of peptic ulcer. *Br. Med. J.*, **1**, 719–29, 786–93

20. Greibe, J. *et al.* (1977). Longterm prognosis of duodenal ulcer: follow-up study and survey of doctor's certificates. *Br. Med. J.*, **2**, 1572–4

21. Editorial (1985). *Lancet*, **1**, 23–4

22. Coggon, D., Lambert, P. M. and Langman, M. J. S. (1981). Twenty years of hospital admissions for peptic ulcer in England and Wales. *Lancet*, **1**, 1300–4

23. Fineberg, H. V. and Pearlman, L. A. (1981). Surgical treatment of peptic ulcer in the United States. *Lancet*, **1**, 1305–7

24. Bateson, M. C. (1984). *Lancet*, **2**, 621–4

25. Bouchier, I. A. D. (1983). *Br. Med. J.*, **1**, 415–6

26. Barker, D. J. P. *et al.* (1979). *Br. Med. J.*, **2**, 1389–92

27. Langman, M. J. S. (1979). *The Epidemiology of Chronic Digestive Diseases.* (London: Arnold)

28. Holland, C. and Heaton, K. W. (1972). *Br. Med. J.*, **3**, 672–5

29. Wenckert, A. and Robertson, B. (1966). *Gastroenterology*, **50**, 376–82

30. Plant, J. C. D. *et al.* (1983). *Lancet*, **2**, 249–51

31. Waller, S. L. and Misiewicz, J. J. (1969). *Lancet*, **2**, 753–6

32. Manning, A. P. *et al.* (1978). *Br. Med. J.*, **2**, 653–4

33. Ritchie, J. and Truelove, S. C. (1979). *Br. Med. J.*, **1**, 376–8

34. Truelove, S. C. (1984). *Ulcerative Colitis.* (Update PGC Series) (London: Update)

35. Parks, T. G. (1969). *Br. Med. J.*, **4**, 639–45

36. Oakley, W. G., Pyke, D. A. and Taylor, K. W. (1978). *Diabetes and its Management.* (Oxford: Blackwell)

37. Commission on Classification of the Terminology of Epilepsy (1981). *Epilepsia*, **22**, 489–501

38. Shorvon, S. D. (1984). *Epilepsy.* (Update PGC Series) (London: Update)

39. Office of Health Economics (1975). *Multiple Sclerosis.* (London: OHE)

40. McAlpine, D. and Compston, M. D. (1952). *Q. J. Med.*, **21**, 135

41. Percy, A. K. *et al.* (1971). *Arch. Neurol.*, **25**, 105

42. Office of Health Economics (1972). *Migraine.* (London: OHE)

43. Waters, W. E. (1974). *Epidemiology of Migraine.* (Bracknell: Boehringen Ingelheim)

44. *Social Trends 1985.* (1985). (London: HMSO)

45. Robinson, S., Golden, J. and Bradley, S. (1983). *A Study of the Role and Responsibilities of the Midwife.* (London: Nursing Education Research Unit/Chelsea College)

46. *On the State of the Public Health.* (London: HMSO)

47. Doll, R. and Peto, R. (1982). *The Causes of Cancer.* (Oxford: Oxford UP)

INDEX